Progress in Epileptic Disorders
Volume 4

**Progress in Epileptic Spasms
and West syndrome**

Progress in Epileptic Disorders
International Advisory Board

Aicardi Jean, *France*
Arzimanoglou Alexis, *France*
Baumgartner Christoph, *Austria*
Brodie Martin, *UK*
Cross Helen, *UK*
Duchowny Michael, *USA*
Elger Christian, *Germany*
French Jacqueline, *USA*
Glauser Tracy, *USA*
Gobbi Giuseppe, *Italy*
Guerrini Renzo, *Italy*
Hirsch Edouard, *France*
Kahane Philippe, *France*
Luders Hans, *USA*
Meador Kimford, *USA*
Moshé Solomon L., *USA*
Noachtar Soheyl, *Germany*
Noebels Jeffrey, *USA*
Palmini André, *Brazil*
Perucca Emilio, *Italy*
Pitkanen Asla, *Finland*
Ryvlin Philippe, *France*
Scheffer Ingrid, *Australia*
Schmitz Bettina, *Germany*
Schmidt Dieter, *Germany*
Serratosa José, *Spain*
Shorvon Simon, *UK*
Tinuper Paolo, *Italy*
Thomas Pierre, *France*
Tuxhorn Ingrid, *Germany*
Wolf Peter, *Denmark*

Progress in Epileptic Disorders
Volume 4

Progress in Epileptic Spasms and West syndrome

Franco Guzzetta
Bernardo Dalla Bernadina
Renzo Guerrini

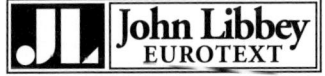

ISBN: 978-2-74-200655-7
ISSN: 1777-4284
Vol. 4.

Published by
Éditions John Libbey Eurotext
127, avenue de la République, 92120 Montrouge, France
Tél. : 01 46 73 06 60
Site internet : http://www.jle.com

John Libbey Eurotext
42-46 High Street
Esher, Surrey
KT10 9KY
United Kingdom

© 2007, John Libbey Eurotext. All rights reserved.

Unauthorized duplication contravenes applicable laws.
Il est interdit de reproduire intégralement ou partiellement le présent ouvrage sans autorisation de l'éditeur ou du Centre Français d'Exploitation du Droit de Copie, 20, rue des Grands-Augustins, 75006 Paris.

Contents

Nosological aspects of West syndrome
    R. Riikonen 1

West syndrome revisited
    G. Avanzini, F. Panzica, S. Franceschetti 15

Infantile spasms and West syndrome: anatomo-electroclinical patterns and etiology
    R. Guerrini, S. Pellacani 23

Epileptic spasms: interictal patterns
    B. Dalla Bernardina, E. Fontana, E. Osanni, R. Opri, F. Darra 43

Epileptic spasms: ictal patterns
    F. Vigevano, P. Montaldo, N. Specchio, L. Fusco 61

Spasms outside West syndrome
    G. Gobbi, D. Frattini, A. Boni, E. Della Giustina, G. Bertani 71

New paediatric behavioural and electrophysiological tests of brain function for vision and attention to predict cognitive and neurological outcomes
    J. Atkinson 83

Developmental features in West syndrome
    T. Deonna, H. Chappuis, D. Gubser-Mercati, A.-L. Ziegler, E. Roulet-Perez 115

West syndrome: epilepsy-induced neuro-sensory disorders and cognitive development
    F. Guzzetta 131

Surgical treatment of West syndrome
    H. T. Chugani, E. Asano, S. Sood 143

The medical treatment of infantile spasms
    G. Coppola, A. Pascotto 153

Foreword

Since its first description (1841) the identity of West syndrome was thoroughly investigated and is now recognized as an epileptic syndrome in infancy (ILAE Task Force).

West syndrome has become a paradigmatic model of an epileptic syndrome causing neurological deterioration (epileptic encephalopathy) and the object of a number of studies aimed at understanding the complex relationships between an epileptic disorder and neurodevelopment. Although the symptomatic triad (peculiar electrographic findings named hypsarrhythmia, brief tonic spasms, and arrest of psychomotor development) that characterizes the syndrome suggests a unique pathogenetic mechanism, causal heterogeneity heavily influences syndrome variability in terms of neurodevelopment, treatment choices, management and, possibly, electroclinical semiology. Important insights may arise for that might help developing models of epileptic encephalopathies in the basic sciences. However, a more immediate benefit may arise for clinicians in everyday practice.

A group of clinical researchers recently met in Rome to discuss hot points concerning infantile spasms and West syndrome. Their contributions were collected and are presented in this book that we hope will contribute to the progress of knowledge of this paradigmatic epileptic disorder.

Franco Guzzetta
Bernardo Dalla Bernardina
Renzo Guerrini

Nosological aspects of West syndrome

Raili Riikonen

Children's Hopital, University of Kuopio, Finland

■ What is West syndrome?

West syndrome is defined as the combination of infantile spasms, hypsarrhythmia, and cognitive regression. The spasms are usually resistant to conventional antiepileptic drugs. The typical syndrome has its onset between 3 and 7 months of age and seldom after the age of one year. Now, however, it is known that there is a great variability of the features. Any feature of this classical triad may be missing.

The incidence of West syndrome has been estimated to vary between 1.6 to 4.3 per 10 000 live births. It has not changed during the past 30 years (Riikonen, 1995).

In his letter to the Lancet, Dr West described the characteristic spasms and noted an association with developmental retardation (West, 1841). Gibbs and Gibbs (1952) first described the EEG pattern commonly seen in infants with infantile spasms, and gave the pattern of hypsarrhytmia its name.

In this review the following topics are presented:
A. Up-to-date classification.
B. Is the syndrome related to a heterogenous array of causes? If so, how?
C. Is the syndrome definition based on age-related mechanisms?
D. How can it be distinguished from earlier or subsequent epileptic encephalopathies?
E. How should late onset or persistent infantile spasms be classified?

■ Up-to-date classification

Infantile spasms are classified as generalized epilepsies according the International Epilepsy Classification (Commission on Classification and Terminology of the International League Against Epilepsy, 1989). In 2001 a revised proposal was developed because "there have been considerable advances in the understanding of the pathophysiology and anatomy of epileptic seizures and disorders" (ILAE Commission report). This classification has been presented as being dynamic and flexible and will be revised periodically. In the future genetic classification of certain epileptic syndromes might also be possible.

Is the classification important for WS?

Classification is important for diagnostic and therapeutic studies of West syndrome. The diagnostic work-up should always be undertaken using pre-defined criteria.

Definitions of key terms

1. Epileptic seizure type: ictal event with unique pathophysiological mechanisms and anatomic substrate, to replace the earlier classification which is based entirely on phenomenology *(new concept)*.

2. Epileptic syndrome: unique epilepsy condition, more than just the seizure type *(changed concept)*.

3. Epileptic encephalopathy: epilepsy contributes to progressive disturbance in cerebral function *(new concept)*.

4. Epileptic disease: pathologic condition with a single well-definied etiology, *i.e.* single gene *(new concept)*.

The prevalence estimate of episodic events, syndromes and diseases in childhood is seen in *Figure 1*.

Three studies (al-Rajeh et al., 1990; Loiseau et al., 1990; Manomani and Tan, 1999) looked at the proportion of infantile spasms among all cases of epilepsy, in both children and adults. All reported low values (1-3%) reflecting the fact that infantile spasms rarely persist beyond early infancy.

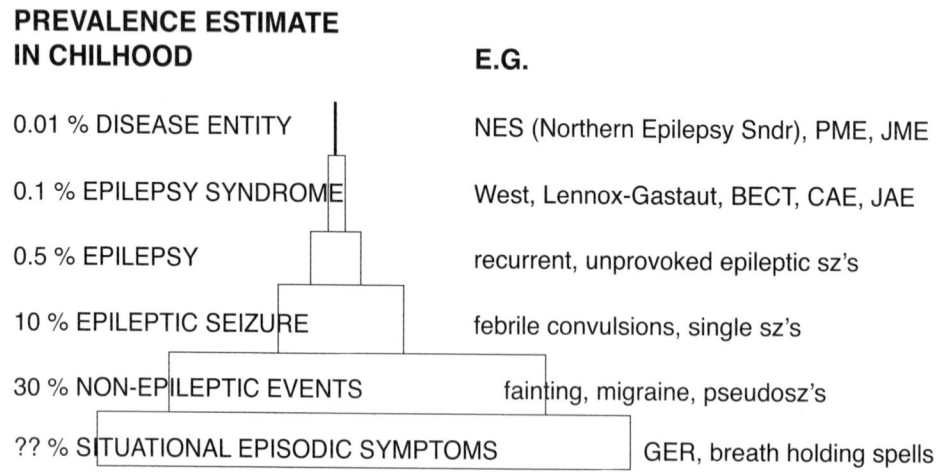

Figure 1. Prevalence estimate of episodic symptoms, syndromes and diseases in childhood.
Published by permission of Acta Universitatis Tamperensis. Eriksson K. Academic dissertation 1998; p. 119.
BECT: Benign childhood epilepsy with centrotemporal spikes. CAE: Childhood absence epilepsy. GER: gastroesophageal reflux. JME: Juvenile myoclonic epilepsy. PME: Progressive myoclonus epilepsy. sz's: seizures.

■ The revised up-to date classification 2001

The diagnostic classification of ILEA Commission report 2001 is divided into five levels:

Level I: Ictal phenemology

Level II: Epileptic seizure type

Level III: Epilepsy syndrome

Level IV: Etiology

Level V: Impairment

Level 1: Ictal phenomenology:

Description of the ictal event, using the standardized Glossary of Descriptive Terminology

What is the relation of West syndrome to this level?

West syndrome: ictal spasms: (flexor, extensor, mixed or subtle type)

Detailed description of the onset and localization of the ictal event is useful for candidates for surgical treatment.

Level 2: Epilepsy seizure type

Seizure types have been divided into

A. Self limited and

B. continuous seizures (status epilepticus)

Self-limited seizures can be divided into

a) generalized and b) focal seizures (localizalized)

What is the relation of West syndrome to seizure type?

West syndrome: Clinical spasms associated with epileptiform EEG: epileptic spasms.

West syndrome: Intermediate between epilepsy with repeat seizures, and status epilepticus. In West syndrome there are seizures but no interictal period because the EEG is continuously abnormal.

Epileptic spasms are seen also in other conditions such as in Ohtahara syndrome, periodic spasms and focal spasms (Gobbi et al., 1987; Ohtsuka et al., 2001; Caraballo et al., 2003). Epileptic spasms may occur after remission of infantile spasms at any age (Camfield et al. 2003).

Level 3: Epileptic syndromes and related conditions

There are a number of epileptic syndromes. In *Table I* are the syndromes of early childhood in order of age at presentation.

Table I. Epileptic syndromes of childhood by order of age appearance

Benign familial neonatal seizures
Early myoclonic encephalopathy
Ohtahara syndrome
"Migrating partial seizures of infancy"
West syndrome
Benign myoclonic epilepsy of infancy
Benign infantile seizures (nonfamilial)
Dravet's syndrome
HH syndrome
Benign childhood epilepsy with centrotemporal spikes
Early-onset benign occipital epilepsy (Panayiotopoulos type)
Late onset childhood occipital epilepsy (Gastaut type)
Epilepsy with myoclonic absences
Epilepsy with myoclonic-astatic seizures
Lennox-Gastaut syndrome
Landau-Kleffner syndrome
Epilepsy with continuous spike-and-waves during slow-wave sleep (other than LKS)
Childhood absence epilepsy
Progressive myoclonic epilepsies
Idiopathic generalized epilepsies with variable phenotypes
Reflex epilepsies
Autosomal dominant nocturnal frontal lobe epilepsy
Familial temporal lobe epilepsies
Generalized epilepsies with febrile plus
Familial focal epilepsy with variable foci
Symptomatic focal epilepsies

West syndrome is an epileptic syndrome consisting of :

a) clinical spasms, usually in clusters

b) hypsarrhythmia or "modified" hypsarrhythmia (variant of hypsarrhythmia) on interictal EEG

c) onset usually under two years of age

The term hypsarrhythmia means an EEG pattern of irregular, diffuse, asymmetric, high-voltage slow waves, interspersed with sharp waves and spikes, distributed randomly throughout scalp recordings (see Dalla Bernardina et al., p. 43).

Modified hypsarrhytmia may be defined as some preservation of background activity, synchronous bursts of generalized spike-wave activity, asymmetry, focality or multifocality.

The term "modified hypsarrhythmia" has not been clearly defined in the literature. EEG is nearly always abnormal and is currently the only laboratory test that provides information for diagnosing infantile spasms.

By using this classification, West syndrome corresponds to ILAE four-level system: level 1. ictal: clinical spasms, level 2. epilepsy type: epileptic spasms, and level 3. syndrome: infantile spasm syndrome.

■ Is the syndrome related to heterogenous array of causes? If so, how?

Can a heterogenous condition be regarded as a single entity?

Syndromes of infantile spasms can be classified according to etiology as symptomatic (80%) and cryptogenic (20%). In the symptomatic group, there is a pre-peri or postnatal history of a disease and a predisposing etiology can be identified. In the cryptogenic group there is a normal prior development, normal imaging and absence of etiological factors. This group has a probably symptomatic etiology; underlying factors remain unknown. It has been recommended that the term cryptogenic should be replaced by the more precise term "probably symptomatic."

The idiopathic group (5%) refers to a pure functional cerebral dysfunction. Genetic factors play an important role.

According to this definition proposal, the cryptogenic cases will later exhibit evidence of persistent brain dysfunction while idiopathic cases recover completely with no residual brain dysfunction. This definition is based on the later outcome, and cannot be confirmed with certainty at the time of diagnosis on the basis of history and presenting features.

The terms idiopathic and cryptogenic have been used as synonyms of each other in some studies. The reader must carefully consider the specific criteria used in each study before assuming that the results of various investigations can be safely compared.

The etiology determines greatly the characteristics of the clinical and EEG pattern.

- Most causes are related to non-progressive cortical lesions.
- Patients classified as cryptogenic had symmetric hypsarrhythmia in up to 94 percent in the study by Donat and Rho (1994).
- The focal features, including focal spikes and slow waves, indicate the presence of an hemispheric lesion. Focal EEG changes preceed 30% of infantile spasms (Riikonen, 1982; Yamamoto et al., 1988).
- More recently Gaily et al. 2001 reported that asymmetrical ictal fast activity occurred significantly more often in symptomatic than in cryptogenic cases.
- The presence of subtle spasms, asymmetric or asynchronous spasms and focal signs suggests a symptomatic etiology (Gaily et al., 1995).
- The age of onset of epilepsy has been suggested to depend on the topography, with the occipital lesions producing spasms earlier than frontal ones (Chugani et al., 1987; Koo and Hwang, 1996; Dulac et al., 1999).

Classification depends heavily on the extent of the investigations performed. Many different disorders damaging the brain seem to be etiological causes of West syndrome.

In one population-based cohort including 208 children with West syndrome, the actual incidence of identified etiologic factors was as follows: 22% of children had brain malformations or malformation syndromes and tuberous sclerosis; insults at birth were the cause in 7%; unknown pre-and/or perinatal factors in 18%, early infections in 4%;

symptomatic neonatal hypoglycemia in 15%, and familial or metabolic cases in 8%. In 18% the cause was cryptogenic (Riikonen, 1995). In spite of decreased perinatal mortality, and decreased incidence of low birth weight infants among the identified cases during the more recent period, the incidence of this disorder did not decline.

At autopsy, two-thirds of the patients with West syndrome have been considered to have epilepsy of embryofetal origin (Meencke and Gerhard, 1985; Jellinger, 1987). Also during epilepsy surgery patients are often found to have microdysgenesis (Vinters et al., 1992, Chugani et al., 1993). In clinical and radiologic series, 20% are found to have malformations.

Neuropathological findings in 38 patients with West syndrome showed that about one half of the lesions were located cortically and the other half subcortically (Riikonen, 2001).

Infantile spasms are a non-specific, although time-limited response and can result from lesions in widespread locations cortical or subcortical, assuming that they are present at the appropriate maturational stage.

Genetics

A number of genetic diseases are encountered in West syndrome *(Table II)*.

Table II. Genetic disorders in West syndrome

Tuberous sclerosis (Riikonen and Simell 1990)
Aicardi's syndrome (Aicardi *et al.* 1965)
Lissencephaly type 1 (Dobyns *et al.* 1984)
PEHO syndrome (Salonen *et al.* 1991)
ARX-gene mutation (clinical picture variable; ranging from cryptogenic to lissencephaly) (Strömme *et al.* 2002)
Familial 4-5% (Riikonen 1987, Dulac *et al.* 1993)
Idiopathic familial (Vigevano *et al.* 1993)

■ Is the syndrome definition based on age-dependent mechanisms?

A specific period of brain maturation is believed to be fundamental to the development of infantile spasms. Infantile spasms usually appear at the age which corresponds to the critical period of maximal brain development. The discrepancy between brain development and age is supported by the following:

– Infantile spasms and hypsarrhythmia tend to disappear with age – there is a natural recovery in 25% (Hrachovy et al., 1991).

– Defective dendritic development, suggesting possible developmental arrest, has been shown at autopsy (Huttenlocher, 1974).

– Glucocorticoids have an accelerating effect on physiological events (enzymes, myelination, neuroblast growth (Palo and Savolainen, 1974; Dunn and Gispen, 1977; Lindholm et al., 1994; Mochetti et al., 1996). ACTH increases the levels of brain NGF in patients with infantile spasms (Riikonen et al., 1997).

- Small-for gestational-age infants are more at risk to develop infantile spasms than average-for-gestational age preterm babies (Riikonen, 1995). It seems that a certain maturation of the brain is needed for infantile spasms to develop.
- It has recently been suggested that early stress (injury or insult) during the critical pre-and perinatal period may increase corticotrophin-releasing factor (CRF) synthesis and activity (Baram, 1993; Brunson et al., 2001; Rho, 2004). This will result in long-term effects. Other pathogenetic theories relate to dysfunction of the brain stem (Satoh et al., 1986) and abnormal cortical-subcortical interaction. Cortical lesions may trigger some subcortical structures (Chugani et al., 1992).

Maturational theory of West syndrome
(Riikonen 1983, Riikonen et al. 1997)

During early development, neurotrophic factors play an important role in the neuronal development and formation of synapses.

Before ACTH therapy, infants with cryptogenic etiology had largely normal levels of nerve growth factor (beta-NGF) in the cerebrospinal fluid. Infants with symptomatic etiology had low levels. Infants with symptomatic, postinfectious etiology had very high levels of NGF (*Figure 2*) (Riikonen et al., 1997). The low levels of NGF might be due to a lack of stimulatory effects. Steroids stimulate neurotrophic factors (Lindholm et al., 1994; Mochetti et al., 1996). Neurons require continuous influx of steroids.

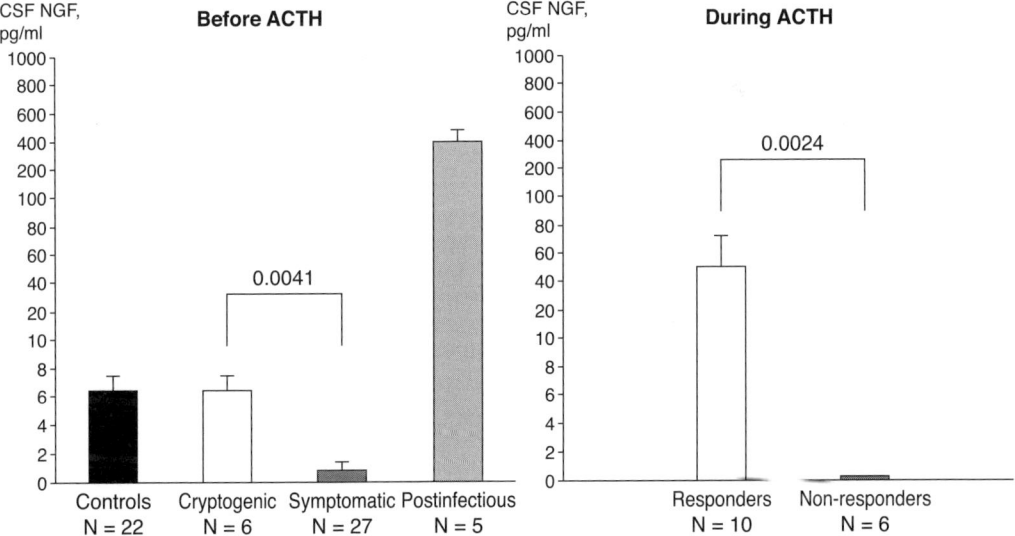

Figure 2. Cerebrospinal fluid beta-nerve growth factor (NGF) levels in 38 infants with West syndrome: before starting ACTH therapy and during the maximal therapy.
Reprinted from *Pediatr Neurology*. Riikonen et al. 1997:17. West's syndrome; Cerebrospinal fluid nerve growth factor and effect of ACTH. pp 22-29. Copyright (2006), by permission from Elsevier.

Cerebrospinal ACTH, measured before therapy, has been in fact lower in children with symptomatic etiology for spasms than with cryptogenic etiology (Riikonen 1996). Highly damaged brain is unable to synthetize NGF and adequately to react to stress, and unable to undergo normal maturational with pruning of synapses. We have shown low CSF NGF in patients with a symptomatic etiology.

There might be an imbalance between inhibitory factors (GABA, NGF) and excitatory factors (glutamate and nitritates/nitrites) (Airaksinen et al., 1992; Riikonen, 1996; Vanhatalo and Riikonen, 2001). The therapeutic action of ACTH could be explained by potentiation of nerve growth factor stimulating effect leading to a balance between inhibitory (nerve growth factor) and excitatory (nitrite/nitrate) factors.

Early stress theory was also discussed by Baram (1993). Infants with infantile spasms have abnormal CSF ACTH and cortisol, markers of the "central" stress-neuroendocrine system (Baram et al., 1995).

Altered maturational processes could possibly explain why so many seemingly independent etiological factors lead to the same clinical syndrome.

■ How to distinguish West syndrome from earlier or subsequent epileptic encephalopathies

Benign myoclonus of early infancy may closely mimic infantile spasms but the EEG is normal (Lombroso and Fejerman, 1977). *Benign myoclonic epilepsy* which has a favourable outcome, is also often misdiagnosed as infantile spasms but the EEG shows generalized spike-waves occurring in brief bursts during the early stages of sleep (Dravet et al., 1985). Syndromes, closely related to West syndrome include *early myoclonic encephalopathy* (Aicardi and Goutiers, 1978), *early infantile epileptic encephalopathy* (Ohtahara et al. 1987) and the syndrome of *periodic, lateralized spasms* (Gobbi et al., 1987). The two former syndromes both have a burst-suppression pattern on EEG. The three syndromes include patients with very serious brain pathology and poor outcome.

Epileptic encephalopathy

A particular group of usually age-related and extremely intractable epilepsies characterized seem to generalized "minor" seizures and massive epileptic EEG abnormalities, both of which cause deterioration in mental and cognitive functions in addition to the pre-existing intellectual deficit due to an organic brain lesion. An organic lesion can be found in 80% in West syndrome.

Encephalopathies closely related to West syndrome, such as early myoclonic encephalopathy, early infantile encephalopathy and Lennox-Gastaut syndrome are briefly presented.

Early myoclonic encephalopathy (EME)

Is characterized by onset before the age of 3 months:
– fragmentary myoclonus from onset, eratic partial seizures;
– massive myoclonic or tonic spasms;
– EEG: suppression-burst (S-B);
– severe course; lack of psychomotor development, death < 1 year of age frequent familial cases.

Early-infantile encephalopathy (Ohtahara syndrome, OS)

– onset before 3 months of age;
– frequent tonic spasms;
– suppression – burst pattern (waking and sleeping states);
– heterogeneous etiology and pathology;
– severe psychomotor retardation;
– often evolution to West syndrome at age 4-6 months.

Lennox-Gastaut syndrome (LGS)

– early childhood;
– multiple and complex seizures: tonic spasms, atonic-astatic attacks, absence, myoclonus;
– EEG: slow background, slow 1-2.5 Hz spike-wave complexes and generalized fast rhythms especially in slow sleep.

There is a transition between the syndromes (*Figure 3*).

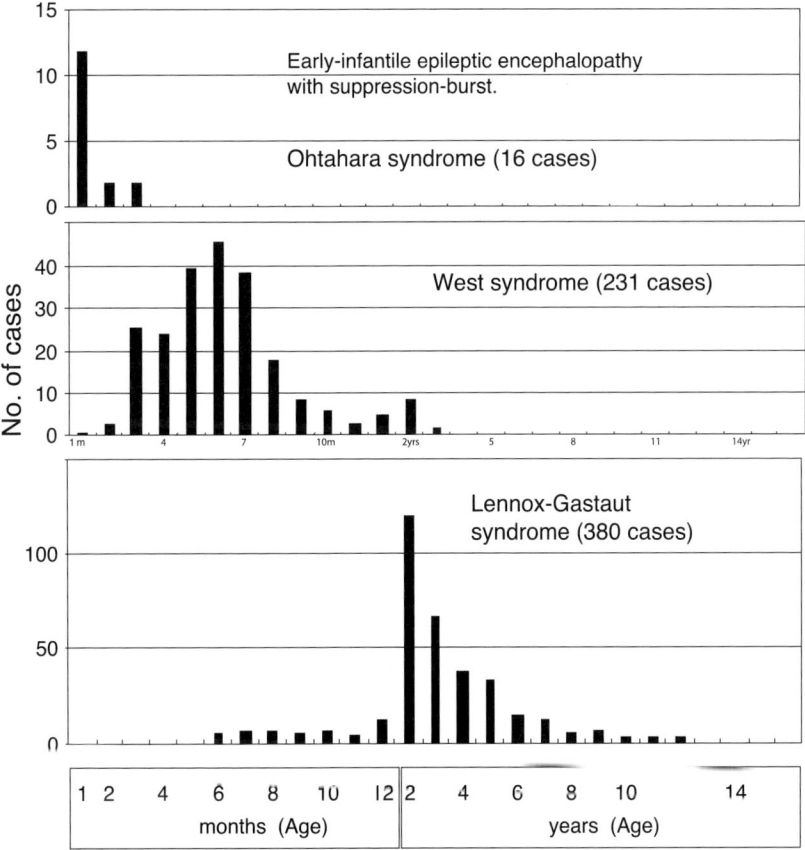

Figure 3. Age at onset of "minor" seizures in three types of age-dependent epileptic encephalopathy.
Reprinted from *Brain Dev* 2002. Yamatogi Y and Ohtahara S. Early infantile epileptic encephalopathy with suppression-bursts; its overview referring to our 16 cases 2002; 24: 13-23. Copyright (2006), with permission from Elsevier.

Early infantile encephalopathy will often evolve into West syndrome. West syndrome evolves in about one-quarter of the patients into Lennox-Gastaut syndrome, which is an important differential diagnosis for patients more than one year of age. Transition between the syndromes suggests an overlapping pathophysiology. It might be an age-specific reaction to various non-specific exogenous brain insults.

Early myoclonic encephalopathy and Ohtahara syndrome have common characteristics: very early onset with frequent "minor" seizures and S-B pattern. In early myoclonic encephalopathy the suppression-pattern persists up to 4 years. Early myoclonic encephalopathy has no specific EEG evolution.

In Ohtahara syndrome EEG evolution is a distinctive feature. Characteristic age-dependent evolution from Ohtahara syndrome to West syndrome, and further from West syndrome to Lennox-Gastaut syndrome in some, preceed concomitantly with EEG transition S-B to hypsarrhythmia and at age of 3 months to diffuse slow-waves at around age one. S-B disappears at around the age of 6 months *(Figure 4)*.

The differentation bewween the four syndromes is seen in *Table III*.

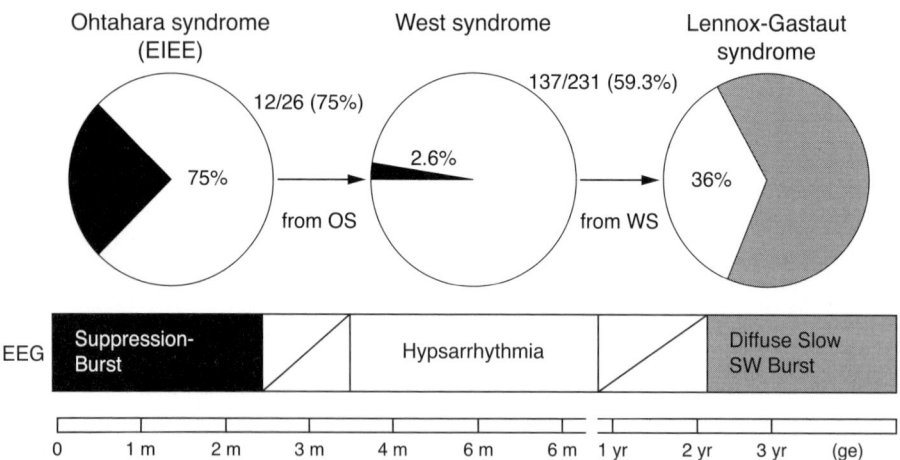

Figure 4. Transition between the syndromes. Characteristic age-dependent evolution from Ohtahara syndrome to West syndrome and further from West syndrome to Lennox-Gastaut syndrome: EEG shows transition from burst-suppression pattern at age of 3 months, to diffuse slow-wave activity at around the age of one. Suppression burst disappears with 6 months.
Reprinted from *Brain Dev* 2002. Yamatogi Y and Ohtahara S. Early infantile epileptic encephalopathy with suppression-bursts; its overview referring to our 16 cases 2002; 24: 13-23. Copyright (2006), with permission from Elsevier.

Tonic spasms are seen in West syndrome and in Ohtahara syndrome. In Ohtahara syndrome tonic spasms are seen in series, also in the sleeping state. The response to ACTH may be good in West syndrome, but poor in others.

Interictal EEG shows S-B in the two early encephalopathies (early myoclonic encephalopathy and Ohtahara syndrome), hypsarrhythmia in West syndrome and is diffuse in Lennox-Gastaut syndrome.

Table III. Differentation between early myoclonic epilepsy (EME), Ohtahara syndrome (OS), West syndrome and Lennox-Gastaut syndrome

	Ohtahara EIE	WS	Lennox-Gastaut
Age	Early infancy	Infancy	Early childhood
Diverse seizures	±	–	++
Tonic spasms	±	+	–
Response to ACTH	Poor	Good	Poor
Interictal	S-B	HYPS	Diffuse

S-B = suppression burst pattern. Hyps = hypsarrhythmia.

■ How to classify the delayed onset of infantile spasms or their persistence after the first years of life?

The spasms may be delayed in onset (Talwar et al. 1995; Sotero de Menezes and Rho 2002). In 2% to 6% of patients the spasms begin after the age of one year (Hrachovy and Frost 1989,, Bednarek et al. 1998).

Late onset epileptic spasms do not figure in the international classification of epilepsy, some authors even disagree with the labelling as infantile spasms. Late onset epileptic spasms merely represent a late variant of the classical West syndrome. The reason for the late onset may be a peri- or postnatal lesion (in contrast, for early onset prenatal lesion). Also, the location of the lesion in the cortex determines in part the age of onset. Lesions affecting the posterior half of the brain often generate at an earlier age than those affecting the anterior half (Chugani et al., 1993; Koo and Hwang, 1996; Dulac et al., 1999).

The spasms usually disappear by 3-4 years of age. However, most patients continue to have significant developmental delay. In the large Finnish series, infantile spasms were persistent in 4/124 patients during a follow-up up of 8-10 years (Riikonen, 1996). Recently, Sotero de Menzes and Rho (2002) described 26 children with West syndrome that did not resolve in infancy. Epileptic spasms continued up to 17 years. Severe disorders, like severe perinatal asphyxia were often associated.

The persistence of the spasms could be explained by delayed maturation of the cortex in patients with severe brain lesions. Early pre-or postnatal stress postnatally may cause the brain to be unable to produce nerve growth factors for inhibitory synaptic maturation (Riikonen, 1997).

■ Conclusions

West syndrome is an age-dependent epileptic syndrome. It is suggested that the phenomenon is related to a deficit in the modulation of neurotransmitters at a specific period of brain *maturation* which is believed to be fundamental to the development of infantile spasms.

There is a *great variability of various features* including age of onset, characteristic spasms, psychomotor development, and EEG activity.

The *heterogenous etiology* greatly determines the characteristics of the clinical and EEG pattern. Focal abnormalities may precede or follow infantile spasms. They indicate a cortical pathology.

Early myoclonic encephalopathy and Ohtahara syndrome may precede West syndrome. They are distinguished by a burst-suppression pattern in EEG. The onset of West syndrome may be delayed after age of one year. Lennox-Gastaut epilepsy may follow West syndrome in 25% of cases.

Acknowledgements

This study was financially supported by Kuopio University, Kuopio, Finland.

References

Aicardi J, Goutieres F. Encephalopathie myoclonique neonatale. *Rev EEG Neurophysiol* 1978; 8: 99-01.

Aicardi J, Lefebure J, Lerique-Koechlin A. A new syndrome. spasms in flexion,callosal agenesis,ocular abnormalities. *Electroenceph Clin Physiol* 1965; 19: 609-10.

Airaksinen E, Tuomisto L, Riikonen R. The concentrations of GABA, 5-HIAA and HVA in the cerebrospinal fluid of children with infantile spasms and the effects of ACTH treatment. *Brain Dev* 1992; 14; 386-90.

al-Rajeh S, Abomelha A, Awada A, Bademosi O, Ismail H. Epilepsy and other convulsive disorders in Saudi Arabia: a prospective study od 1,000 consecutive cases. *Acta Neurol Scand* 1990: 341-45.

Baram T, Mitchell W, Hanson R, Snead O.C.3rd, Horton E. Cerebrospinal fluid corticotrophin and cortisol is reduced in infantile spasms. *Pediatr Neurol* 1995; 13: 108-10.

Baram T. Pathophysiology of massive infantile spasms: perspective on the putative role of the brain adrenal axis. *Ann Neurol* 1993; 33: 231-36.

Bednarek N, Motte J, Soufflett C, Plouin P, Dulac O. Evidence of late-onset infantile spasms. *Epilepsia* 1998; 39: 55-60.

Brunson K, Khan N, Eghbal-Ahmadi M, Baram T. Corticotropin acts directly on amygdala neurons to down-regulate corticotropin-releasing hormone gene expression. *Ann Neurol* 2001; 49: 304-12.

Camfield P, Camfield C, Lortie A, Darwish H. Infantile spasms in remission may reemerge as intractable epileptic spasms. *Epilepsia* 2003: 1592-95.

Caraballo H, Fejerman N, Dalla Bernadina B *et al*. Epileptic spasms in clusters without hypsarrhytmia in infancy. *Epileptic Disord*. 2003; 5: 109-13.

Chugani H, Shewmon D, Shields W *et al*. Surgery for intractable infantile spasms: neuroimaging perspectives. *Epilepsia* 1993; 3: 764-71.

Chugani H, Phelps M, Mazziotta J. Positron emission tomography of human brain functional development. *Ann Neurol* 1987; 22: 487-97.

Chugani H, Shewmon A, Sankar R, Chen B, Phelps M. Infantile spasms: II. Lenticular nuclei and brain stem activation on positron emission tomography. *Ann Neurol* 1992; 131: 212-9.

Commission on Classification and Terminology of the International League Against Epilepsy. Proposal for revised classification of epilepsies and epileptic syndromes. *Epilepsia* 1989; 34: 389-99.

Dobyns W, Stratton R, Greenberg F. Syndromes with lissencephaly. I: Miller-Dieker and Norman-Roberts syndromes and isolated lissencephaly. *Am J Med Genetics* 1984; 18: 509-26.

Donat J, Lo W. Assymmetric hypsarrhythmia and infantile spasms in West syndrome. *J Child Neurol* 1992; 9: 290-6.

Dravet C, Giraud N, Bureau M, Roger J, Gobbi C, Dalla Bernadina B. Benign myoclonus of early infancy or benign non-epileptic infantile spasms. *Neuropediatrics* 1986; 17: 33-8.

Dulac O, Chiron C, Robain O et al. Infantile spasms: a pathophysiological hypothesis. In: Nehlig A, Motte J, Moshe S, Plouin P. Editors. *Childhood epilepsies and brain development*. London: John Libbey, 1999: 93-102.

Dulac O, Feingold J, Plouin P, Chiron C, Pajot N, Ponsot G. Genetic predisposition to West syndrome *Epilepsia* 1993; 34: 732-7.

Dunn A, Gispen W. How ACTH acts on the brain? *Biobehaviour Reviews* 1977; 1: 15-23.

Eriksson K. Severe epilepsies, epileptic syndromes, and status epilepticus. Prevalence, classification, associated neuroimpairment and choices of treatment. Academic dissertation, Acta Universitatis Tamperensis 590; 1998.

Gaily E, Shewman D, Chugani H, Curran J. Asymmetric and asynchronous infantile spasms. *Epilepsia* 1995; 36: 873-82.

Gaily E, Liukkonen E, Paetau R, Rekola R, Granström M L. Infantile spasms: diagnosis and assessment of treatment response by video-EEG. *Dev Med Child Neurol* 2001: 43: 658-67.

Gibbs F, Gibbs E. *Atlas of electroencephalography*. Cambridge, Mass. Addison-Wesley, 1952.

Gobbi G, Bruno L, Pini A, Giovanardi Rossi P, Tassinari C. Periodic spasms: an unclassified type of epileptic seizure in childhood. *Dev Med Child Neurol* 1987; 27: 766-75.

Hrachovy R, Frost J. Infantile spasms. *Pediatric Clincs of North America* 1989; 36: 311-29.

Hrachovy R, Glaze D, Frost Jr J. A retrospective study of spontaneous remission and long-term outcome in patients with infantile spasms. *Epilepsia* 1991; 32: 212-21.

Huttenlocher P. Dendritic development in neocortex of children with mental defect and infantile spasms. *Neurology* 1974; 24: 203-10.

ILEA Commission Report. A proposed diagnostic scheme for people with epileptic seizures and with epilepsy: Report of the ILEA task force on classification and terminology. *Epilepsia* 2001; 42: 796-803.

Jellinger K. Neuropathological aspects of infantile spasms. *Brain Dev* 1987; 9: 349-57.

Koo B, Hwang P. Localization of focal cortical lesions influences age of onset of infantile spasms. *Epilepsia* 1996; 37: 1068-71.

Lindholm D, Castren M, Hengerer B, Leingärtner A, Castren E, Thoenen H. Glucocorticoids and neurotrophin gene regulation in the nervous system. *Ann NY Acad Sc USA* 1994; 746: 195-02.

Loiseau J, Loiseau P, Guyot M, Duche B, Dartigues J-F, Aublet B. Survey of seizure disorders in the French Southwest. I. Incidence of epileptic syndromes. *Epilepsia* 1990; 31: 391-6.

Lombrosco C, Fejerman N. Benign myoclonus of early infancy. *Ann Neurol* 1: 138-43.

Manonmani V, Tan C. A study of newly diagnosed epilepsy in Malaysia. *Singapore Med J* 1999; 40; 32-5.

Meencke H, Gerhard C. Morphological aspects of aetiology and the course of infantile spasms (West syndrome). *Neuropediatrics* 1985; 16: 59-60.

Mocchetti I, Spiga G, Hayes V, Isackson P, Colangelo A. Glucocorticoids differentially increase nerve growth factor and basic fibroblast factor expression in the rat brain. *J Neurosci* 1996; 16: 2141-8.

Ohtahara S, Ohtsuka Y, Yamatogi Y, Oka E. The early infantile encephalopathy with suppression-burst: developmental aspects. *Brain Dev* 1987; 9: 371-6.

Ohtahara syndrome; its overview referring to our 16 cases. *Brain Dev* 2002; 24: 13-23.

Ohtsuka Y, Kabayashi K, Ogino T, Oka E. Spasms in clusters in epilepsies other than typical West syndrome. *Brain Dev* 2001; 23: 473-81.

Palo J, Savolainen H. Effect of high doses of synthethic ACTH on the rat brain. *Brain Res* 1974; 70: 313-20.

Rho J. Basic science behind the catastrophic epilepsies. *Epilepsia* 2004; 45 (suppl 5): 5-11.

Riikonen R, Simell O. Tuberous sclerosis and infantile spasms. *Dev Med Child Neurol* 1990; 32: 203-9.

Riikonen R, Söderström S, Vanhala R, Ebendal T, Lindholm D. West's syndrome: Cerebrospinal fluid nerve growth factor and effect of ACTH. *Pediatric Neurology* 1997; 17: 224-9.

Riikonen R. Decreasing perinatal mortality: unchanged infantile spasm morbidity. *Dev Med Child Neurol* 1995; 37: 232-8.

Riikonen R. Epidemiological data of West syndrome in Finland. *Brain Dev* 2001; 23: 539-41.

Riikonen R. How do cryptogenic and symptomatic infantile spasms differ? Review of biochemical studies in Finnish patients. *J Child Neurol* 1996a; 11: 383-8.

Riikonen R. Infantile spasms in siblings. *J Ped Neurosci* 1987; 3: 235-44.

Riikonen R. Infantile spasms: some new theoretical aspects. *Epilepsia* 1983; 24: 159-68.

Riikonen R. Long-term outcome of West syndrome: a study of adults with a history of infantile spasms. *Epilepsia* 1996b; 37: 367-72.

Salonen R, Somer M, Haltia M, Lorenz M, Norio R. Progressive encephalopathy with edema, hypsarrhythmia, and optic atrophy (PEHO syndrome). *Clin Genetics* 1991; 39: 287-93.

Satoh J, Mizutani T, Horimatsu Y. Neuropathology of the brainstem in age-dependent epileptic encephalopathy – especially in cases of infantile spasms. *Brain Dev* 1986; 8: 443-9.

Sotero de Menezes M, Rho J: Clinical and electrographic features of epileptic spasms persisting beyond the second year of life. *Epilepsia* 2002; 43: 623-30.

Strömme P, Mangelsdorf M, Scheffer I, Gecz J. Infantile spasms, dystonia, and other x-linked phenotypes caused by mutations in Aristaless related homeobox gene, ARX. *Brain Dev* 2002; 24: 266-8.

Talwar D, Baldwin M, Hutzler R, Griesemer D. Epileptic spasms in older children: persistence beyond infancy. *Epilepsia* 1995; 36: 151-5.

Vanhatalo S, Riikonen R. Nitric oxide metabolites, nitrates and nitrites in the cerebrospinal fluid in children with West syndrome. *Epilepsy Res* 2001; 146; 3-13.

Vigevano F, Fusco L, Cusmai R, Claps D, Ricci S, Milani L. The idiopathic form of West syndrome. *Epilepsia* 1993; 34; 743-6.

Vinters H, Fisher R, Cornford M *et al.* Morphological substrates of infantile spasms: studies based on surgically cerebral tissue. *Childs Nerv Syst* 1992:8: 8-17.

West W. On a pecular form of infantile convulsions. *Lancet* 1841: I: 724-5.

Yamamoto N, Watanabe K, Negoro T *et al.* Partial seizures evolving to infantile spasms. *Epilepsia* 1988; 29: 3-40.

West syndrome revisited

Giuliano Avanzini, Ferruccio Panzica, Silvana Franceschetti

Istituto Nazionale Neurologico C. Besta, Milano, Italy

Infantile Spasms (ISs), *i.e.* short tonic contractions involving the axial muscles and proximal limb segments, have been identified as epileptic phenomena since they were first described by *West (1841)* as "a peculiar form of infantile convulsions" that typically occur in early infancy (usually between the third and twelfth month) and have a remarkable tendency to cluster with a quasi periodic time course. These features are so typical that the term of IS (properly referred to a seizure type) is frequently used as a synonym for West syndrome and related disorders, which typically present with seizures in series (Commission on pediatric epilepsy of the International League Against Epilepsy, 1992). The association of infantile spasms with "chaotic" interictal EEG discharges (hypsarrhythmia, Gibbs and Gibbs, 1952) and impairment of psychomotor development was considered the distinctive presentation of the relatively common infantile epileptic encephalopathy known as West syndrome (West, 1841; Gastaut et al., 1964, Duncan, 2001). The inclusion of developmental delay as a definition criterion is disputed, as at the onset of spasms it is likely to be assessed unreliably; moreover, the presentation of spasms in cluster is considered a highly characteristic feature of West Syndrome.

According to the consensus of experts participating in the so called West Delphi group, West syndrome is a subset of the syndrome of infantile spasms (ISs), which is defined as an epilepsy syndrome characterized by clinical spasms that usually occur in cluster, its onset is usually within the first year of life (rarely in children older that 2 years). The most characteristic EEG feature associated with ISs is hypsarrhythmia (usually interrupted during the clinical attack of epileptic spasms), which is however not found in all cases nor throughout the clinical course of the condition. Many potential etiologies or associated conditions exist. ISs are often associated with developmental arrest or regression (Lux and Obsborne, 2004).

Spasms are very brief, with the muscle contraction lasting from some hundreds of milliseconds to a few (usually 1-2) seconds and are typically associated with a "diamond-like" EMG pattern with fast incrementing/decrementing muscle contraction.

Polygraphic studies (Kellaway et al., 1979) and extensive Video-EEG recordings (Donat and Wright, 1991) have shown that more than one type of spasm may occur in the same infant, and that the motor phenomena may be asymmetric (Kellaway et al., 1979). A considerable body of literature concerning unusual presentations of ISs has been accumulated over the past years, suggesting that fragmentary motor phenomena, often presenting with unilateral or focal features (Donat and Wright, 1991; Watanabe et al., 1994; Gaily et al., 1995) may replace (or occur with) typical spasms. Furthermore, episodes of behavioral "arrest" accompanying or replacing the spasms have been reported as ictal phenomena (Kellaway et al., 1979). There are various reasons for classifying these disparate ictal symptoms and massive spasms as homogeneous expressions of early infantile epilepsies. Indeed, both massive ictal phenomena more properly called ISs, on which the original definition of West was based, and fragmentary, sometimes focal motor fits or even ictal "arrests" can occur in the same series; moreover, series of both subtle and massive motor phenomena can occur, and individual fits can increase in strength over time, often terminating with a "decreasing" trend. This sequence might suggest a common physiopathological substrate for each individual ictal event making up the series. In addition, long-lasting electrographic changes (i.e. a marked decrease in interictal activity or focal slowing) often precede the onset and persist between the individual ictal events, until the end of a series. This may suggest that the spasms (and/or their subtle substitute) take place during the course of a long lasting change in the physiological (or physiopathological) state of the brain, which is interrupted by periodic phenomena.

Within a series, the interval between spasms may be regular or irregular, often over a period of many minutes. The maximum frequency of spasms within a series evaluated by Kellaway et al. (1979) was 13 per minute, and the maximum number of spasms making up a series was 125. The duration of a series may vary in the same infant, and an isolated spasm can occasionally occur in an infant who usually has seizures in series. Spasms predominantly occur soon after arousal, although they can also appear during wakefulness and sleep.

The typical ictal EEG change associated with each spasm is a complex and variable waveform including slow and/or sharp transients, variably associated with attenuation and/or short discharges of fast activity (Kellaway et al., 1979) lasting from one to a few seconds. Several studies have shown that the ictal EEG event can consist of a fragment of the above-mentioned patterns, and that fast activity, alone or superimposed over background attenuation, may be the only seizure pattern. In the study of Kellaway et al. (1979), characteristics of the ictal EEG events did not strictly correlate with the type of spasm (flexor, extensor or mixed), but "arrest" and asymmetrical seizures were typically associated with attenuation and fast activity discharges.

■ Pathophysiology

In spite of the extensive neurophysiological and neuropathological studies, the physiopathological substrate of spasms and the location of their primary generator are still unclear and controversial. Some authors (Kellaway et al., 1983; Hrachovy and Frost, 1989) have proposed a brainstem generator as the only source of spasms, on the basis that a dysfunction of brainstem nuclei (*i.e.* pontine reticular formation) can generate spasms interfering with the cortico-spinal afferences controlling spinal reflexes. According to this model, both ictal and interictal phenomena (*i.e.* hypsarrhythmia) may be due to an abnormal input to cortical (or thalamic) structures. Some evidence supporting this model comes from the occasional observation of pathological changes affecting the pontine nuclei in infants with West syndrome (Satho et al., 1986), and from electrophysiological evidence of altered brainstem auditory potentials, suggesting a local dysfunction (Kaga et al., 1982). In addition, the specific involvement of axial structures has been suggested by biochemical evidence indicating specific serotonergic neurotransmission impairment (Colemann, 1971; Langlais et al., 1991).

On the contrary, a considerable body of clinical and neuropathological evidence supports the primary involvement of cortical structures in the generation of both ictal and interictal patterns that characterize the epileptic encephalopathies presenting with spasms. In particular it has been stressed that prominent focal or diffuse cerebral damage involving the cerebral cortex is evident in many cases of infant symptomatic epilepsies presenting with spasms, and many cases of IS have been attributed to neuropathological lesions specifically involving the neocortex such are cortical malformations (Kang et al., 2006) or acquired disruptive lesions, phakomathoses, etc. Moreover, several reports describe the therapeutic effect of surgical resection of localized cortical lesions (Uthman et al., 1991; Shields et al., 1992). In addition, it is known that callosotomy may interrupt a bilateral hypsarrhythmia, suggesting that a cortico-cortical pathway through the corpus callosum is involved in the diffuse expression of interictal activity in West syndrome (Pinard et al., 1993). The corticogenic hypothesis is further supported by the frequent observation that subtle lateralized motor fits presenting in series (and subsequently evolving into massive spasms), as well as asymmetric spasms, can be time locked with a contralateral ictal EEG discharge thus suggesting a focal cortical origin (Watanabe et al., 1994; Gaily et al., 1995).

We studied 18 infants with cryptogenic (n = 6) or symptomatic (n = 12) ISs with repeated awake and sleep Video-EEG and polygraphic recordings (Panzica et al., 1999). In our series the EMG spasm patterns had a relatively homogeneous time course in all of the infants, consisting of a gradual increase in the muscle contraction, which reached a maximum after 540 ± 360 ms, followed by a gradual decrease (total duration $1,470 \pm 890$ ms). The spasms were categorized as symmetric in 12 cases and asymmetric in other 5 cases; the location of the motor phenomena was strictly unilateral in only one case. The lateral eye version, accompanying the spasms in seven cases, was never found to precede the onset of the tonic muscle contraction. The signal deflection of the EOG traces started at the same time as the contraction or followed it after 90-114 ms. However, in three of these cases, a few episodes of only ictal eye deviation did precede the spasm series. No other behavioral ictal phenomena were detected on the video-EEG before or after the spasms.

The autoregressive spectral analysis of the 500 ms EEG epochs preceding spasm onset revealed in 13 of the 18 cases included in the study the presence of a short discharge of fast activity restricted to a narrow frequency band. The fast discharge peaked at 17.5 ± 2.1 Hz, with rather low inter-hemispheric coherence values (0.52 ± 0.17) and asymmetric amplitude on homologous EEG derivations (*Figure 1*). It persisted briefly

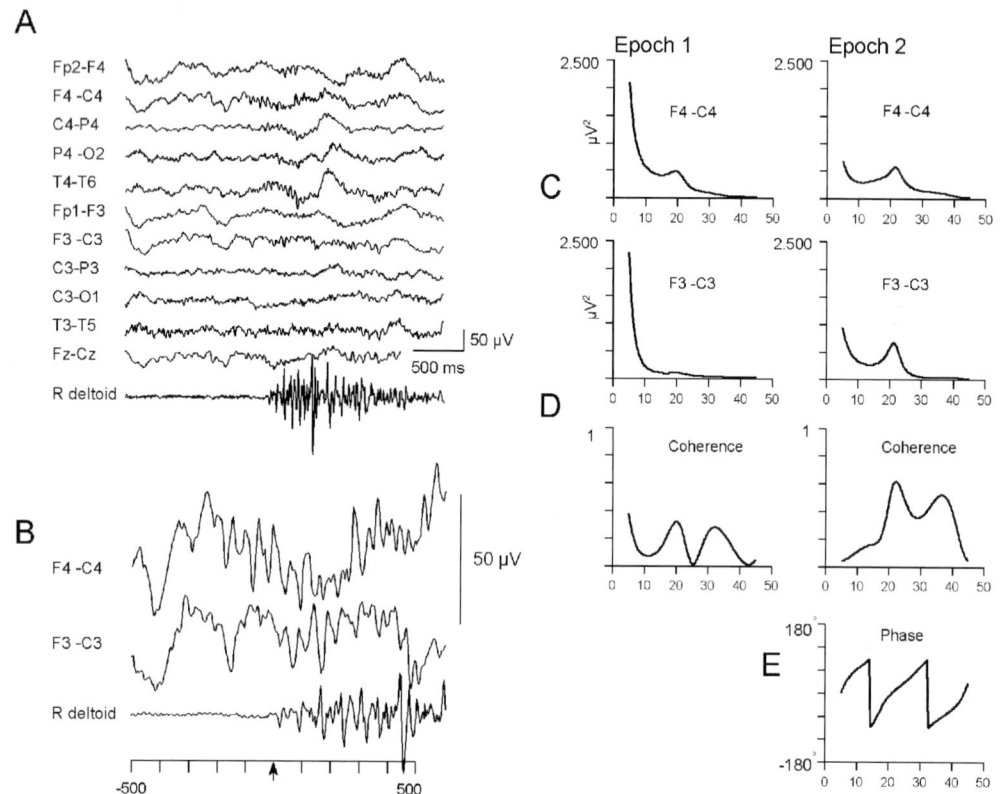

Figure 1. EEG sample relating to an individual spasm recorded in an infant with cryptogenic West syndrome.
Visual inspection of the EEG ictal event indicated that the amplitude of the fast activity discharge was higher on the right hemisphere, with an apparent fronto-central onset preceding the spasm (see the high magnification display in B, where the arrow indicates spasm onset). AR analysis of the 500 ms epoch preceding the spasm detected a clear peak of 19.2 Hz activity from the right F-C derivation (C), which was just detectable from the homologous contralateral derivation. Inter-hemispheric coherence (D) of fast activity was low (0.32) before spasm onset, and increased to 0.62 during the following 500 ms epoch, and the estimated inter-hemispheric time difference was 6.5 ms (E).
From Panzica *et al.* 1999 with permission.

after spasm onset, reaching a higher coherence value (0.71 ± 0.16). The inter-hemispheric time difference, estimated in those cases with the coherence values significantly different from zero, ranged from 9.1 to 14.3 ms (11.4 ± 1.9 ms) in the epoch preceding spasm onset.

The asymmetric EEG pattern (mainly consisting of a rhythmic burst of fast activity), which consistently preceded both symmetric and asymmetric spasms, led us to a localized cortical origin of the ictal discharge giving rise to the spasms. In fact, it has been demonstrated that EEG activities in beta range are commonly generated by the cortical network under physiological conditions (Steriade *et al.*, 1996), and are comparable with the commonly described EEG patterns characterizing focal seizures in infants and adults (Yamamoto *et al.*, 1987; Luna *et al.*, 1989; Connolly *et al.*, 1995; Commission on Classification and Terminology of the International League Against Epilepsy, 1989). Interestingly, rhythmic discharges of action potentials in the beta range have been found to characterize the firing behavior of subsets of regular spiking and intrinsically bursting neocortical pyramidal neurons recorded in both adult (Silva *et al.*, 1991; Tseng and Prince, 1993) and immature experimental animals (Franceschetti *et al.*, 1998). In addition, the rather long inter-hemispheric time difference of fast activity (more than 10 ms) convincingly suggests the hypothesis of a secondary transfer of rhythmic EEG activity from a primary epileptogenic area to the homologous contralateral region, in agreement with the criteria proposed by Gotman (1981, 1983) and supported by Kobayashi *et al.* (1992) by both experimental and clinical evidence. More recently, preliminary evidence collected in our laboratories indicate the consistency between the side of earliest appearance of EEG fast activity associated with infantile spasms, and the onset of local EEG discharges occurring during the follow up in 10 infants (Panzica *et al.*, 2006). It can be also hypothesized that a cortical generator requires a subcortical pacemaker in order to synchronize homologous neocortical regions. Neither of these hypotheses excludes the possibility that brainstem (*i.e.* pontine) structures may be recruited from unilateral descending input to generate bilateral involvement in the tonic contraction-giving rise to the spasm. Furthermore, the assumption that a cortical ictal discharge can trigger an "archaic" brainstem circuit to sustain the motor phenomena of spasms appears to be the simplest way of explaining the massive behavioral pattern characterizing this seizure type, which is reminiscent of Moro reflex (Gobbi *et al.*, 1987) or startle reactions (Brown *et al.*, 1991).

Along this line, the possibility that subcortical structures may produce periodic flexor or extensor spasms because of dishinibition from cortical control impaired by diffuse cortical dysfunction (Dulac *et al.*, 1994) should also be taken into account.

The assumption of a localized cortical origin for spasms is further supported by the fact that in our cases with asymmetric spasms, the greater power associated with the fast activity peak was invariably contralateral to the side of the body on which the motor ictal phenomena were stronger, but was always ipsilateral to lateralizing interictal EEG patterns (*e.g.* "consistent" focus accompanying hypsarrhythmia) and/or neuroradiologically detectable hemispheric damage in infants with symmetric or asymmetric spasms. The idea of a localized onset of ISs have been sustained because the lateralized location of spasm associated slow waves (Kobayashi *et al.*, 2005) and because a clear local onset detected by means of invasive recordings in infants and children submitted to presurgical evaluation (Asano *et al.*, 2005).

As far as the age-dependent mechanisms responsible for the peculiar semeiology of IS, an interesting insight has been provided by experimental studies on N-methyl-D-aspartate (NMDA) – induced seizures in developing rats (Mareš and Velišek, 1992; Kabowa *et al.*, 1999). The result of NMDA administration at 7th, 12th, 15th and 18th postnatal days clearly show important developmental changes in seizure patterns. Relevant to the present topic is the observation that flexion seizures (reminiscent of human ISs), associated with electrocorticographic flattening, show a marked age-dependence. They could in fact be observed reliably only between the 7th and the

18th day old animals, a time in which the immature glutamatergic transmission in the neocortex undergoes important changes leading to a mature organization which is attained around the end of the third postnatal week (Avanzini et al., 1992; Bugard and Hablitz, 1993).

Immature glutamate-mediated excitatory postsynaptic potentials (EPSPs) are particularly prolonged because of a NMDA mediated component which is less sensitive to the voltage-dependent Mg^{2+} block than in adults (Avanzini et al., 1992; Bugard and Hablitz, 1993)

Although the reason why the immaturity of NMDA receptors result in flexor rather than extensor type of seizures is still unclear, Mareš and Vališek's (1992) observation could be accounted for by the marked facilitation of the NMDA-mediated component shown by the above quoted experiment in the same range of rat postnatal ages.

In conclusion more than a century and half after the unsurpassed description of William West on his own son, the intimate nature of IS remains elusive. The two main questions i.e. what is the pathophysiological mechanism underlying this peculiar type of seizures and why it is electively activated during a rather narrow developmental window are in fact largely unanswered. Upon these two points, every advance in designing strategies aimed at preventing or discontinuing IS course is based.

From the existing information, we can draw only some limited conclusions.

First of all, the classification of ISs among the generalized seizures (i.e. seizures "in which the first clinical change indicate initial involvement of both hemisphere" (Commission on classification and terminology of the International League against Epilepsy, 1981) is questionable in view of the evidence of a lateralized onset. In general one would rather define the IS pattern as "diffuse" rather than generalized.

Second, the similarity of the IS with Moro reflex suggests that spasms are generated by some archaic circuit hypothetically located in the brainstem either through an excitatory or disinhibitory mechanism. In the first instance, the hypothesis is that the discharge, wherever originated, gets access to the brainstem generator thus triggering it; in the second case, the discharge involving the cortex would disrupt its inhibitory control on brainstem thus "liberating" the archaic reflex. In either case, IS expression is obviously related to the same developmental window in which Moro reflex is observed, their further persistence being accounted for by plastic changes that tend to stabilize the circuit over its physiological term. Although partly speculative these hypotheses can suitably account for many clinical aspects of IS syndrome including the peculiar profile of its pharmacological sensitivity, which differentiates them from all other types of epilepsies.

The most serious gap in our understanding of ISs is the lack of information on the mechanisms that orient different epileptogenic factors (such as cerebral dysplasia, phakomathoses or some primary etiological mechanism defined as cryptogenic) toward this always severe type of infantile epileptic encephalopathy. In the absence of fully reliable animal models of IS all the potential of the exploration techniques usable in the clinical setting should be employed to advance our knowledge thus improving our ability to counteract this harmful infantile epilepsy.

References

Asano E, Juhasz C, Shah A, Muzik O, Chugani DC, Shah J, Sood S, Chugani HT. Origin and propagation of epileptic spasms delineated on electrocorticography. *Epilepsia* 2005; 46 (7): 1086-97.

Avanzini G, Franceschetti S, Panzica F, Buzio S. Age-dependent changes in excitability of rat neocortical neurons studied in vitro. In: Molecular neurobiology of epilepsy, eds. J. Engel, C. Wasterlain, A. Cavalheiro, U. Heinemann and Avanzini. *Epilepsy Res* 1992; (suppl) 9: 95-105.

Brown P, Rothwell JC, Thompson PD, Britton TC, Day BL, Marsden CD. The hyperekplexias and their relationship to the normal startle reflex. *Brain* 1991; 114: 1903-28.

Bugard EC, Hablitz JJ. Developmental changes in NMDA and non-NMDA receptor-mediated synaptic potentials in rat neocortex. *J Neurophysiol* 1993; 69: 230-40.

Colemann M. Infantile spasms associated with 5-hydroxytryptophan administration in patients with Down's syndrome. *Neurology* 1971; 21: 911-9.

Commission on Classification and Terminology of the International League Against Epilepsy. Proposal for revised classification of epilepsy, epileptic syndromes. *Epilepsia* 1989; 30: 389-99.

Commission on classification and terminology of the International League Against Epilepsy. Proposal for revised clinical and electroencephalographic classification of epileptic seizures. *Epilepsia* 1981; 22: 489-501.

Commission on pediatric epilepsy of the International League Against Epilepsy. Workshop on infantile spasms. *Epilepsia* 1992; 33: 195.

Connolly MB, Langill L, Wong PK, Farrell K. Seizures involving the supplementary area in children: a video-EEG analysis. *Epilepsia* 1995; 36: 1025-32.

Donat JF, Wright FS. Unusual variants of infantile spasms. *J Child Neurol* 1991; 6: 313-8.

Dulac O, Chiron C, Robain O, Pouin P, Jambaque II, Pinard JM. Infantile Spasms: a pathophysiological hypothesis. *Semin Pediatr Neurol* 1994; 1 (2): 83-9.

Duncan R. Infantile spasms: the original description of Dr West in 1841. *Epileptic Disord* 2001; 3 (1): 47-8.

Franceschetti S, Sancini G, Panzica F, Radici C, Avanzini G. Postnatal differentiation of firing properties and morphological characteristics in layer V pyramidal neurons of the sensory motor cortex. *Neuroscience* 1998; 83: 1013-24.

Gastaut H, Roger J, Soulayrol R, Pinsard N. *Encepalopathie myoclonique infantile avec hypsarythmie (Syndrome de West)*. Paris: Masson, 1964.

Gibbs FA, Gibbs EL. *Atlas of electroencephalography, Vol. II, Epilepsy*. Cambridge: Addison-Wesley, 1952.

Gaily EK, Shewmon DA, Chugani HT, Curran JG. Asymmetric and asynchronous infantile spasms. *Epilepsia* 1995; 36: 873-82.

Gobbi G, Bruno L, Pini A, Giovanardi Rossi P, Tassinari CA. Periodic spasms: an unclassified type of epileptic seizures in childhood. *Develop Med and Child Neurol* 1987; 29: 766-75.

Gotman J. Interhemispheric relations during bilateral spike-and-wave activity. *Epilepsia* 1981; 22: 453-66.

Gotman J. Measurement of small time differences between EEG channels: method and application to epileptic seizure propagation. *Electroenceph Clin Neurophysiol* 1983; 56: 501-14.

Hrachovy RA, Frost JD. Infantile spasms: a disorder of the developing nervous system. In: *Problems and concepts in developmental neurophysiology*, eds. P. Kellaway & J.L. Noebels, 1989: 131-47. Baltimore: J. Hopkins University Press.

Kabova R, Liptakova S, Slamberova R, Pometlova M, Velisek L. Age-specific N-methyl-D-aspartate-induced seizures: perspectives for the West syndrome model. *Epilepsia* 1999; 40 (10): 1357-69.

Kaga K, Marsh RR, Fukuyama Y. Auditory brainstem responses in infantile spasms. *J Pediatr Otorhinolaryngol* 1982; 4: 57-67.

Kang HC, Hwang YS, Park JC, Cho WH, Kim SH, Kim HD, Park SK. Clinical and electroencephalographic features of infantile spasms associated with malformations of cortical development. *Pediatr Neurosurg* 2006; 42 (1): 20-7.

Kellaway P, Hrachovy RA, Frost JD jr., Zion T. Precise characterization and quantification of infantile spasms. *Ann Neurol* 1979; 6: 214-8.

Kellaway P, Frost JD, Hrachovy RA. Infantile spasms. In: *Antiepileptic drug therapy in pediatrics*, eds. P.D. Morselli, C.E. Pippenger & J.K. Penry, 1983: 115-36. N.Y.: Raven Press.

Kobayashi K, Ohtsuka Y, Oka E, Ohtahara S. Primary and secondary bilateral synchrony in epilepsy: differentiation by estimation of inter-hemispheric small time differences during short spike-wave activity. *Electroncephal clin Neurophysiol* 1992; 83: 93-103.

Kobayashi K, Oka M, Inoue T, Ogino T, Yoshinaga H, Ohtsuka Y. Characteristics of slow waves on EEG associated with epileptic spasms. *Epilepsia* 2005; 46 (7): 1098-105.

Langlais PJ, Mark LW, Hitoshi Y. Changes in CSF neurotransmitters in infantile spasms. *Pediatr Neurol* 1991; 7: 440-5.

Luna D, Dulac O, Plouin P. Ictal characteristics of cryptogenic partial epilepsies in infancy. *Epilepsia* 1989; 30: 827-32.

Lux AL, Obsoborne JO. A proposal for case definition and outcome measures in studies of infantile spasms and West syndrome: consensus statement of the West Delphi Group. *Epilepsia* 2004; 45: 1416-28.

Mareš P, Velišek L. N-Menthyl-D-aspartate (NMDA)-induced seizures in developing rats. *Developmental Brain Research* 1992; 65: 185-9.

Panzica F, Binelli S, Granata T, Freri E, Visani E, Franceschetti S. Ictal fast EEG discharges in infantile spasms, from onset to outcome. *Clin Neurophysiol* 2006; 117, (suppl 1) S144-145.

Panzica F, Franceschetti S, Binelli S, Canafoglia L, Granata T, Avanzini G. Spectral propertis of EEG fast activity ictal discharges associated with infantile spasms. *Clinical Neurophysiology* 1999; 110: 593-603.

Pinard JM, Delande O, Pluin P, Dulac O. Callosotomy in west syndrome suggest a cortical origin of hypsarrhythmia. *Epilepsia* 1993; 34: 780-7.

Satho J, Mizutani T, Morimatsu Y. Neuropathology of the brainstem in age dependent epileptic encephalopathy especially in cases of infantile spasms. *Brain Dev* 1986; 8: 443-9.

Shields WD, Shewmon DA, Chugani HT, Peacock WJ. Treatment of infantile spasms: medical or surgical? *Epilepsia* 1992; 33 (suppl 4): s21-s26.

Silva LR, Amitai Y, Connors BW. Intrinsic oscillations of neocortex generated by layer 5 pyramidal neurons. *Science* 1991; 251: 432-5.

Steriade M, Amzica F, Contreras D. Synchronization of fast (30-40 Hz) spontaneous cortical rhythms during brain activation. *J Neurosci* 1996; 16: 392-417.

Tseng GF, Prince DA. Heterogeneity of rat corticospinal neurons. *J Comp Neurol* 1993; 335: 92-108.

Uthman BM, Reid SA, Wilder BJ, Andriola MR, Beydoun AA. Outcome for West syndrome following surgical treatment. A case report. *Epilepsia* 1991; 32: 668-71.

Watanabe K, Toshiko H, Tamiko N, Kousaburo A, Norihide M. Focal spasms in clusters, focal delayed myeliantion, and hypsarrhythmia: unusual variant of West Syndrome. *Pediatr Neurol* 1994; 11: 47-9.

West WJ On a peculiar form of infantile convulsion. *Lancet* 1841; I: 724-5.

Yamamoto N, Watanabe K, Negoro T, Takaesu E, Aso K, Fuune S, Takahashi I. Complex partial seizures in children: ictal manifestations and their relation to clinical course. *Neurology* 1987; 37: 1379-82.

Infantile spasms and West syndrome: anatomo-electroclinical patterns and etiology

Renzo Guerrini, Simona Pellacani

Child Neurology Unit, Children's Hospital A. Meyer-University of Florence, Via Luca Giordano 13, Firenze Italy

Infantile spasms (IS) are a distinctive form of seizure disorder, mainly observed in infants, during the first year of life, and refractory to conventional antiepileptic drugs. Developmental delay or deterioration and a characteristic EEG pattern (*hypsarrhythmia*), are often associated to infantile spams, configuring *West syndrome*. The seizure type in itself, irrespective from the age and clinical context, is defined as *epileptic spasm* (Dulac *et al.*, 1994) and may rarely occur in childhood or even in adulthood (Egli, 1985; Ikeno *et al.*, 1985; Bednarek *et al.*, 1998; de Menezes and Rho, 2002; Cerullo *et al.*, 1999).

The muscle contraction of infantile spasms has distinctive features. It reaches its maximum more slowly than a myoclonic jerk and decreases in an equally slower way (Fusco and Vigevano, 1993), though it is faster and less sustained than observed in tonic seizures.

■ Electroclinical characteristics

Spasms

Infantile spasms implicate a sudden, generally bilateral, contraction of muscles of the neck, trunk, and extremities. *Flexor spasms* have long been regarded as the hallmark of the syndrome. They consist of a sudden flexion of the head, trunk and legs, which are usually held in adduction. The arms, also in flexion, can be adducted or abducted. Mixed flexorextensor spasms are the most common type. They consist of either flexion of the neck, trunk, and arms with extension of the legs or, less commonly, flexion of the legs and extension of the arms. *Extensor spasms*, involving an abrupt extension of the neck and trunk, with extension and abduction of the arms, are less common (Lombroso, 1983). Most affected infants have more than one type of spasm.

The intensity of the contractions and the number of muscle groups involved vary considerably both in different infants and in the same infant with different attacks. The spasms may consist of only slight head nodding, upward eye deviation, or elevation and adduction of the shoulders in a shrugging movement. In some cases, the spasms may be so slight that they can be felt but not seen, or they may be clinically unnoticeable even though they are shown on polygraphic recordings (Kellaway et al., 1979). The number of spasms usually is much higher of what is reported by parents (Gaily et al., 2001). The electromyographic tracing in an infantile spasm consists of an abrupt initial contraction lasting less than 2 sec, followed by a more sustained contraction lasting 2 to 10 sec (Kellaway et al. 1979). The second, or tonic, phase may be absent, the spasm being limited to the initial phasic contraction lasting 0.5 sec or less. The contraction may appear diamond-shaped on electromyographic recordings (Fusco and Vigevano, 1993).

In 6 to 8% of cases, the spasms may be asymmetrical or even unilateral (Kellaway et al., 1979; Lombroso, 1983). Asymmetrical spasms are associated with a symptomatic etiology, but unilateral lesions can generate symmetrical attacks. Asymmetrical spasms may occur after a partial seizure (Yamamoto et al., 1988).

Lateralized motor phenomena, including lateral or upward eye deviation and eyebrow contraction, abduction of one shoulder, may sometimes constitute the entire series of spasms or initiate a series which will eventually develop into bilateral phenomena. Such lateralized manifestations are usually accompanied by unilateral or asymmetric ictal EEG changes.

Spasms are characteristically grouped in series or clusters. The clusters consist of a few units to more than 100 individual jerks, 5 to 30 sec apart. The intensity of the jerks in a series may initially wax and wane, not always regularly. Status of infantile spasms has been reported (Coulter, 1986). The number of series is variable from only 1 to 50 or more daily (Lacy and Penry, 1976). Clusters may occur during sleep, usually at the time of awakening or at the transition from slow sleep to REM sleep (Plouin et al., 1987). They are frequent in drowsiness. No obvious precipitating stimuli or circumstances are detectable in most infants. However, self precipitation prompted by complex behaviors is occasionally observed (Guerrini et al., 1992) *(Figure 1)*. Following a series of spasms, the infant may be left exhausted and lethargic. Spasms may change their characteristics becoming more subtle, spontaneously or as effect of treatment. Video-EEG monitoring may be necessary to provide firm evidence that spasms have really disappeared in response to medication (Gaily et al., 2001).

Hypsarrhythmia and the ictal EEG

The hypsarrhythmic EEG is characterized by very high-voltage (up to 500 µV) slow waves, irregularly interspersed with spikes and sharp waves that occur randomly in all cortical areas. The abnormal discharges are not synchronous over both hemispheres, so the general appearance is that of a chaotic disorganization of electrogenesis. Hypsarrhythmia is an interictal pattern observed mainly while the child is awake. During slow sleep, bursts of more synchronous, polyspikes and waves, often appear (Lombroso, 1983). The term "modified hypsarrhythmia" has been used by some

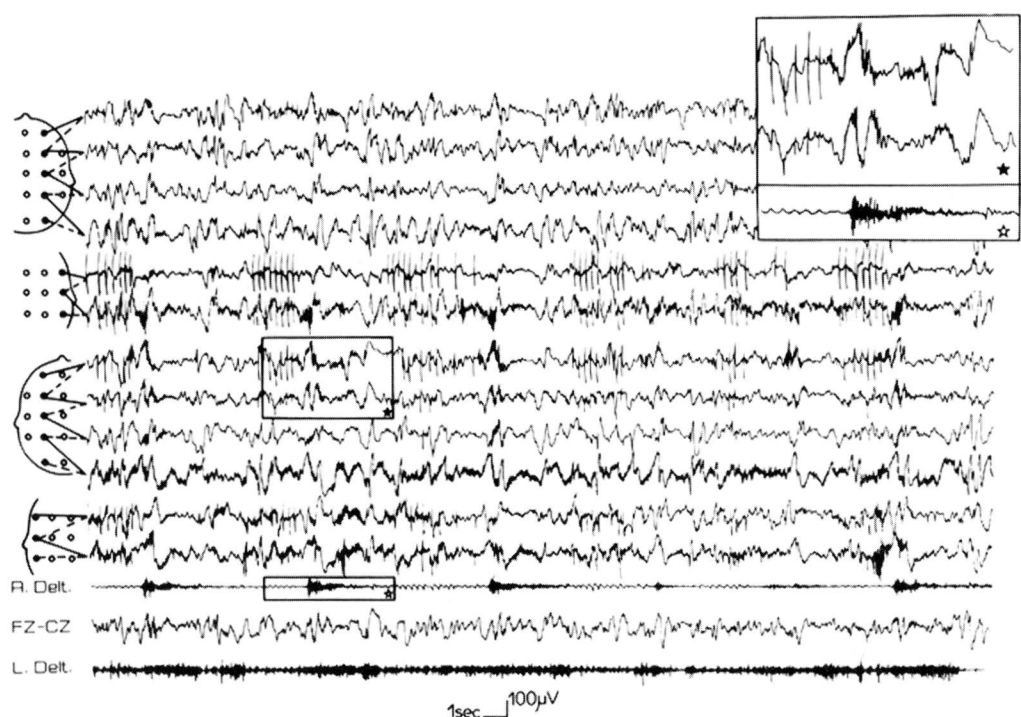

Figure 1. Ictal EEG recording of a series of self induced spasms in a 6 years old boy with severe developmental delay.
Each spasm is triggered by a series of repetitive taps of the right hand on the chin. Rhythmic tapping artifacts precede a triphasic slow wave with superimposed low-voltage fast activity, which is more prominent over the left hemishere and is accompanied by a tonic contraction predominating in the right deltoid (R. Delt). (From Guerrini *et al.*, 1992).

investigators to designate EEG patterns with atypical features, such as relatively preserved background activity, generalized synchronous spike-wave discharges, prominent asymmetry or suppression-bursts (Hrachovy *et al.*, 1984).

It has been suggested that cognitive and behavioral deterioration, which is typical of the syndrome, might result from persistent hypsarrhythmic EEG activity, possibly representing a variant of nonconvulsive status (Dulac, 2001).

Hypsarrhythmia tends to disappear in older children, occasionally even when spasms may still be observed (Hrachovy and Frost, 1989). The tracings may then become normal or exhibit various abnormalities.

Intravenous diazepam may suppress hypsarrhythmia and unmask focal discharges (Dalla Bernardina and Watanabe, 1994).

Ictal EEG patterns are variable; the most common is a high voltage, frontal-dominant, generalized slow-wave transient, with an inverse phase reversal over the vertex, followed by voltage attenuation (Fusco and Vigevano, 1993). Bilateral and diffuse fast rhythms in the b-range (occasionally in (d-band) coincide with the clinical spasm and with the initial part of the low voltage record, which lasts two to 5 sec. In many cases, only voltage attenuation (decremental discharge) may be observed. Spams with a more sustained tonic contraction, likewise tonic seizures, are accompanied by a high-amplitude slow wave, followed by fast activity (Vigevano et al., 2001).

Other ictal patterns include generalized sharp-and-slow wave complexes, generalized slow-wave transients only, or fast rhythms in isolation (Kellaway et al., 1983). Asymmetrical and unilateral spasms are usually associated with contralateral EEG activity, suggesting unilateral damage. After the initial spasms of a series, there may be transient suppression of the hypsarrhythmic pattern, which will not reappear between consecutive spasms. In other cases, hypsarrhythmia resumes between spasms. It has been suggested that disappearance of hypsarrhythmia in the course of a series of spasms might indicate a symptomatic origin, whereas its resumption in between serial spasms would indicate an "idiopathic" condition and carry a favorable prognosis (Dulac, 1997).

Children with severe structural brain abnormalities, such as tuberous sclerosis, Aicardi syndrome or lissencephaly, do not usually have typical hypsarrhythmia. It is likely that only children with less severe brain impairment, and higher chances of a better outcome, are able to generate a typical hypsarrhythmic pattern.

■ Differential diagnosis

A rare condition, termed *benign myoclonus of early infancy*, is characterized by repetitive jerks that closely mimic infantile spasms but are not accompanied by EEG abnormalities and have a spontaneously favorable course (Dravet et al., 1986; Fejerman and Caraballo, 2002). Benign myoclonus, however, although repetitive, never presents with the periodic character of spasms. Another manifestation, called "repetitive sleep starts" (Fusco et al., 1999), often observed in children with spasticity, may closely mimic infantile spasm. These starts might represent a pathological enhancement of hypnagogic jerks, which are cyclically repeated while the infants are falling asleep. Tonic upgaze deviation, repeated in clusters every few seconds for several minutes, may be seen in *benign tonic upward gaze*, occurring in previously normal children between age 6 and 20 months (Guerrini et al., 1998). During the attacks, EEG is normal and the child, who is conscious, may maintain visual fixation by bending the head downwards, a maneuver that produces vertical nystagmus. This is an age-related condition that disappears within 1-2 years from onset. *Compulsive self gratification behavior* (previously termed as *compulsive masturbation*) is a condition that is mainly observed in girls during late infancy or early childhood. Some of the children may present with prolonged episodes of rhythmic contractions of the lower limbs and trunk with eye staring and adducted thighs with an attitude of withdrawal (Guerrini, 2006).

Early forms of myoclonic epilepsy, especially *benign myoclonic epilepsy*, are mistaken for infantile spasms by the inexperienced clinician. The jerks are briefer than spasms and often have a saccadic appearance. Usually, they are not repeated in series, and are accompanied by a short burst of irregular, fast polyspike-wave complexes on a relatively normal background EEG.

Differentiating infantile spasms from the tonic seizures of Lennox-Gastaut syndrome may be difficult, especially when the attacks are in extension and not repeated in clusters.

■ Etiological factors

Infantile spasms have multiple causes, and their pathophysiological mechanism is unknown. Infants with developmental brain abnormalities and those who are small for gestational age are more apt to develop spasms. The *age dependency* of the disorder is notable. Almost all cases have their onset during the first year of life (Chevrie and Aicardi, 1971). Maximum incidence is between 3 and 7 months. Age of onset, however, depends on the proportion of symptomatic *versus* cryptogenic cases in any particular series. It seems that the location of the cortical lesion(s) may influence age at onset. Koo and Hwang (1996) observed that the earliest onset was seen with occipital lesions; whilst frontal lesions were associated with the latest onset. A family history of infantile spasms is only found in about 4% of the cases (Sugai et al., 2001). Familial cases are probably the expression of several genetic disorders, some of which are well characterized, including leukodystrophy (Coleman et al., 1977), tuberous sclerosis (Riikonen, 1984), X-linked lissencephaly and band heterotopia (Guerrini and Carrozzo, 2001a), X-linked mental retardation and infantile spasms due to mutations of the *ARX* gene (Claes et al., 1997; Stromme et al., 1999; Stromme et al., 2002).

Several apparently unrelated phenotypes have been associated with mutations of the *ARX* gene, including syndromes with and without brain malformations. The former include X-linked lissencephaly with abnormal genitalia (XLAG), severe hydrocephalus and Proud syndrome (agenesis of the corpus callosum with abnormal genitalia), while the latter include X-linked infantile spasms (ISS), Partington syndrome, which consists of mental retardation with mild dystonia, and nonspecific X-linked mental retardation (Stromme et al., 2002; Kato et al., 2004). In general, the malformation phenotypes are associated with protein truncation mutations and missense mutations in the homeobox, while the non-malformation phenotypes are associated with missense mutations outside of the homeobox and expansion of the polyalanine tracts. Boys with X-linked infantile spasms due to *ARX* mutations usually have severe developmental delay and may have microcephaly. Onset of spasms is usually early and hypsarrhythmia is frequent (Stromme et al., 2002; Kato et al., 2003), although not constantly reported. Follow-up data on infantile spasms in these patients are not available. A syndrome of early onset infantile spasms, with hypsarrhythmia and severe quadriplegic dyskinesia, in which spasms tend to remit but episodes of status dystonicus complicate the course, has been associated with expansions in the first polyalanine tract of the *ARX* gene (Guerrini et al., in press).

A syndrome with microcephaly and early onset intractable seizures, including spasms with or without hypsarrhythmia, has been associated with mutations of the *CDKL5* gene in girls (Archer et al., 2006). No unique EEG patter seems to be typical for this etiology. The spectrum of clinical manifestations in girls with *CDKL5* mutations appears to be broad and includes multiple seizure types with early onset and features that may overlap with the Rett syndrome (Mari et al., 2005; Scala et al., 2005; Weaving et al., 2004).

A possibly recessive syndrome of early onset infantile spasms, often preceded and followed by other types of seizures, associated with hypsarrhythmia, facial dysmorphism, optic atrophy and peripheral edema, has been reported from Finland as PEHO syndrome (progressive encephalopathy with edema, hypsarrhythmia, and optic atrophy) (Riikonen, 2001). Cases exist outside Finland.

Other genetic disorders are more rare and may be of recessive (Caplan et al., 1992; Fleiszar et al., 1977; Ciardo et al., 2001) or of undetermined nature (Reiter et al., 2000).

Although infantile spasms are traditionally divided into cases of *symptomatic* and *cryptogenic* origin, the meaning of these terms varies among the studies and according to the extent of investigations. The specific nature of the causative lesion also implies a variable prognostic outlook. Most define as symptomatic those cases in which an etiological factor can be clearly identified. Other investigators link symptomaticity to either or both abnormal development prior to the onset of spasms and clinical or imaging evidence of a brain lesion. Cryptogenic spasms, are those for which no cause can be identified, or development was normal before the onset of spasms. In addition, the term *cryptogenic* does not necessarily mean that a lesion is not present; therefore, a difference of nature between cryptogenic and symptomatic cases is not clearly established. A few cases that are not included in the symptomatic group, despite increasingly accurate investigations, may belong to an "idiopathic" group (Dulac et al., 1986; Vigevano et al., 1993). A typical and symmetric and hypsarrhythmic pattern, that reappear between individual spasms during a clusters in a previously normal child would be an electroclinical feature of idiopathic spasms (Plouin et al., 1987). However, these features are not fully reliable (Haga et al. 1995). In spite of these divergences about definitions the distinction between symptomatic and cryptogenic spasms is of great practical significance because a poor prognosis is expected when a structural brain abnormality is present.

Although the infantile spasms have multiple causes and it is often stated that this seizure type are but a response of the immature brain to multiple types of insults. However, some causes are especially likely to result in infantile spasms.

Malformations of the cerebral cortex (or of cortical development, Barkovich et al., 2005) are a well-established cause of infantile spasms and seem to be involved in about 30% of cases (Guerrini and Marini, 2006).

Tuberous sclerosis (TS) is found in 7-25% of the children who present with infantile spasms (Curatolo et al., 2001). On the other hand about 50% of patients with epilepsy and tuberous sclerosis appear to have or have had infantile spasms (Roger et al. 1984) and about 85% of infants with tuberous sclerosis who experience seizures in the first year of life have infantile spasms (Chevrie and Aicardi, 1977). Onset of spasms may be preceded by partial seizures (Chevrie and Aicardi, 1977; Dulac et al., 1996) and a combination of partial seizures and spasms is often observed in the same child *(Figure 2)*. Waking EEGs show multifocal or focal spike discharges and irregular slow

Infantile spasms and West syndrome: anatomo-electroclinical patterns and etiology

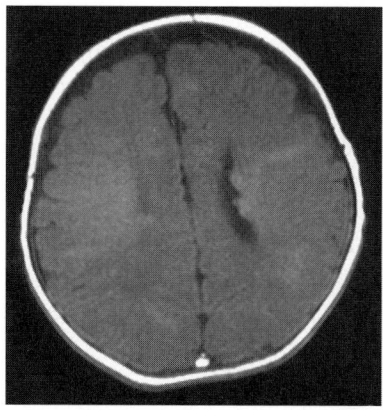

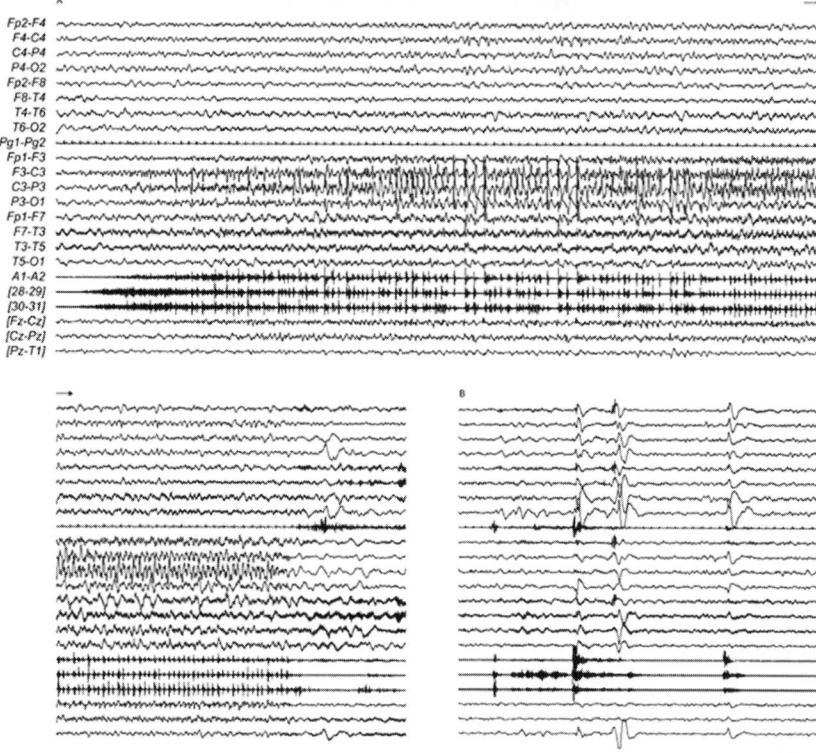

Figure 2. Infantile spasms in tuberous sclerosis.
a. MRI scan of the brain of a 3 months old boy with tuberous sclerosis. Note the subependymal nodules on both sides and multiple areas of high signal intensity, corresponding to cortical tubers.
b. EEG recording of a focal seizure followed by a series of spasms. A and B. Onset of focal ictal activity is observed on the F3-C3 electrode, with spread over neighbouring P3 electrode. An initial tonic contraction is recorded of the right wrist extensor and flexor muscles (28-29 channel and 30-31 channel), followed by activity on the ipsilateral deltoid (A1-A2). Initially arrhythmic and subsequently rhythmic clonic activity is recorded from the same muscles. The whole seizure lasts around 80 seconds and is followed, around 20 seconds after its end by a small series of spasms (B).

focal activity (Dulac et al., 1996; Curatolo, 1996). Abnormalities increase during sleep. Atypical hypsarrhythmia, often asymmetrical, is present in one third of cases. Video-EEG monitoring and analysis of EEG patterns may suggest a focal origin of the spasms (Dulac et al., 1996; Curatolo, 1996). In general, infantile spasms in TS are considered to differ clinically and electro-encephalographically from classical infantile spasms with typical hypsarrhythmia, the main differences including the frequent association with focal seizures, with asymmetric clinical and EEG features and absence of typical hypsarrhythmia.

Cortical tubers are usually well visualized by MRI scan as enlarged gyri with atypical shape and an abnormal signal intensity, mainly involving the subcortical white matter. In the newborn they are hyperintense with respect to the surrounding white matter, on T1 weighted images and hypointense on T2 weighted images. Progressive myelination of the white matter in the older infant gives the tubers an hypointense center on T1 and high signal intensity on T2. The number of tubers is usually multiple. A relationship between location of the tubers and severity of epilepsy has been suggested (Jambaqué et al., 1991, 1993). However, some patients with multiple tubers can be asymptomatic, indicating that the relation between the number and location of tubers is a complex one.

Two genes TSC1 and TSC2 have been identified. The TSC1 gene, mapping 9q34 (van Slegtenhorst et al., 1997) encodes a predicted protein named "hamartin". The TSC2 gene, mapping to 16p13.3 (European Chromosome 16 Tuberous Sclerosis Consortium, 1993) encodes a predicted protein named tuberin. TSC genes are thought to act as tumor suppressors (Carbonara et al., 1994). No obvious phenotypic differences have been found in the families linked to the TSC1 or TSC2 gene mutations, although it has been suggested that patients with TSC1 mutations may have less severe epilepsy and cognitive impairment (Dabora et al., 2001).

The association of infantile spasms with other neurocutaneous syndromes is less clear. West's syndrome has been observed in association with neurofibromatosis, and was said to have a relatively good prognosis (Motte et al., 1993) but the association may be coincidental.

Other brain malformations, especially neuronal migration disorders and focal cortical dysplasia are found with increasing frequency as a cause of infantile spasms (Guerrini et al., 1996; Robain and Vinters, 1994; Dulac et al., 1996). Some malformations have an elective association with infantile spasms. Aicardi's syndrome (Chevrie and Aicardi, 1986) consists of total or partial agenesis of the corpus callosum, chorioretinal lacunae, and infantile spasms that are often asymmetrical and associated with other seizures, especially focal attacks. Neuroimaging demonstrates several brain defects in addition to callosal agenesis or dysgenesis, such as periventricular heterotopia, abnormal gyration, cystic formations around the third ventricle, and gross hemispheric asymmetry (Chevrie and Aicardi, 1986). Unlayered polymicrogyria is observed at histopathology (Guerrini et al., 1993). The EEG is rarely hypsarrhythmic; typically, the tracings are of the so-called split-brain type, with paroxysmal EEG discharges occurring independently over either hemisphere *(Figure 3)*. The onset is often early and may be neonatal. Prognosis is poor; severe developmental delay, neurological abnormalities, and persistence of the spasms are the rule. Aicardi's syndrome is not a familial disorder and should

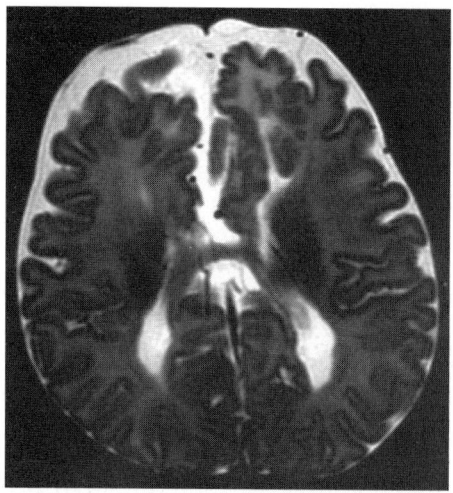
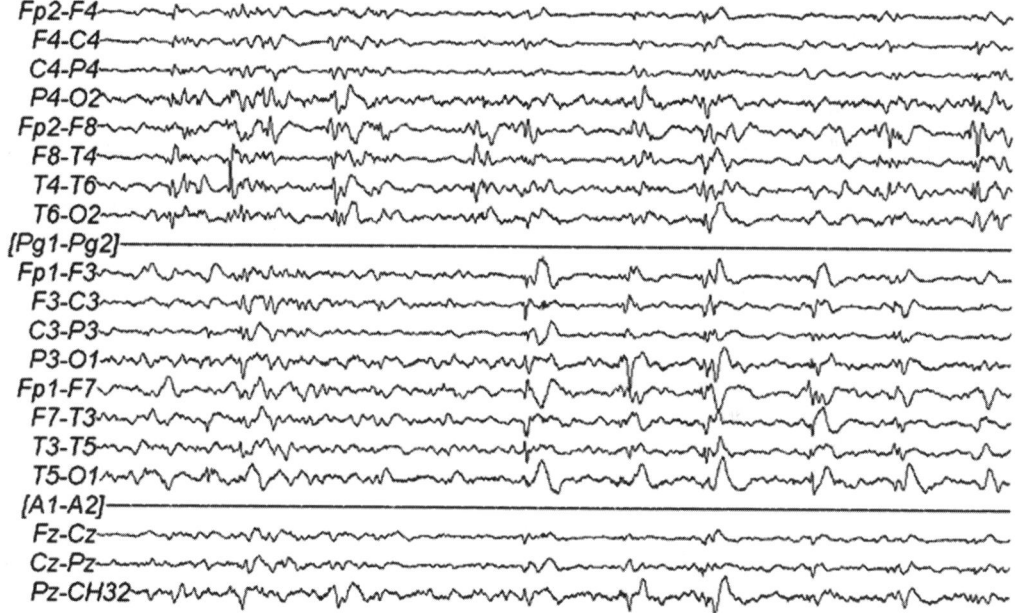

Figure 3. Aicardi syndrome.
a. T2 weighted axial MRI scan of the brain of a 5 months old girl with Aicardi syndrome. Note the hypoplastic corpus callosum with dilated ventricles and an extensive area of polymicrogyria involving the left frontal lobe, especially around the left frontal horn and the anteromesial aspect of the frontal pole. The white matter underlying the polymicrogyric cortex shows high signal intensity
b. Sleep EEG recording of the same girl when aged 9 months. Note the bilateral asynchronous bursts of repetitive spike and wave discharges. (Pg1 is the left deltoid EMG and A1-A2 is the right deltoid).

be separated from the few cases of familial agenesis of the corpus callosum associated with infantile spasms (Cao et al., 1977) and from the rare X-linked lissencephaly with callosal agenesis and ambiguous genitalia, which is only observed in boys with ARX mutations (see above) (Dobyns et al., 1999).

Lissencephaly and pachygyria also have a special relationship with infantile spasms (Dulac et al., 1983; Gastaut et al., 1987; Guerrini and Carrozzo, 2001a, b). Although the diagnosis rests on neuroimaging, interictal EEG shows a highly characteristic pattern with high-amplitude fast rhythms, which may alternate with a mixture of high-amplitude theta and delta rhythms (*Figure 4*) that may suggest slow spike-waves or resemble hypsarrhythmia (Gastaut et al., 1987; Quirk et al., 1993). About 75% of infants with lissencephaly-pachygyria have infantile spasms (Guerrini et al., 1999). However, since studies defining the electroclinical characteristics of agyria pachygyria were published before the distintion between LIS 1-linked and X-linked forms was recognized, it is not known whethere these two main forms have distinctive electroclinical features. Spasms are rarely observed in children with subcortical band heterotopia (Barkovich et al., 1994).

Hemimegalencephaly, which is associated with abnormal gyration and dysplasia of one cerebral hemisphere, is a possible cause of infantile spasms and may be amenable to hemispherectomy (King et al., 1985; Vigevano and Di Rocco, 1990) or hemispherotomy. The EEG tracings may include unilateral fast rhythms and suppression-bursts, or slow spike-wave patterns (Paladin et al., 1989).

Focal cortical *dysplasia* is often detected as abnormal signal on T2-weighted and FLAIR sequences and abnormal folding and thickness of the cortex (Sankar et al., 1995). Thin slices and multiplanar reconstruction (Chan et al., 1998), as well as additional new MRI techniques (Bastos et al. 1999, Eriksson 2001) have enhanced the diagnostic power of neuroimaging. In spite of these increasingly sophisticated techniques, a number of children with infantile spasms harbor small areas of dysplasia that escape recognition by MRI. In addition, in children aged less than 2 years even macroscopic dysplasia may be overlooked, as the typical blurring between gray and white matter may not be apparent due to incomplete myelination (Juhasz et al., 2001). Repeat MRI scan is therefore advised in children with infantile spasms, in whom a first early scan was normal, especially if asymmetric EEG or clinical features are present.

Infantile spasms probably represent the most common seizure type observed in *Down's syndrome* (Stafstrom et al. 1991). In most children, spasms appear without any evidence of additional brain damage (Stafstrom and Konkol, 1994; Silva et al., 1996) and remission is obtained on conventional antiepileptic drugs, ACTH, steroids or vigabatrin, without relapse of seizures or with later onset of a mild age-related generalized seizure disorders (Silva et al., 1996; Nabbout et al., 2001).

Metabolic disorders are not a common cause of infantile spasms. Phenylketonuria is now unlikely to be a cause of infantile spasms in industrialized countries as it is systematically detected by neonatal screening. However, this disorder is electively related to West's syndrome (Poley and Dumermuth, 1968). A hypsarrhythmic EEG occurred in approximately one-third of untreated phenylketonuric patients. Nonketotic hyperglycinemia (glycine encephalopathy) is a rare cause of infantile spasms.

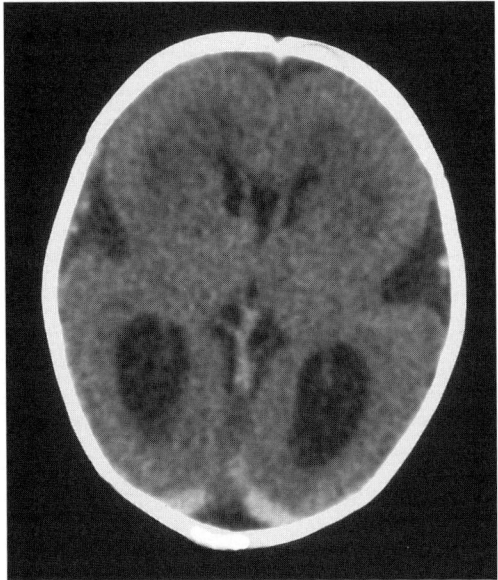

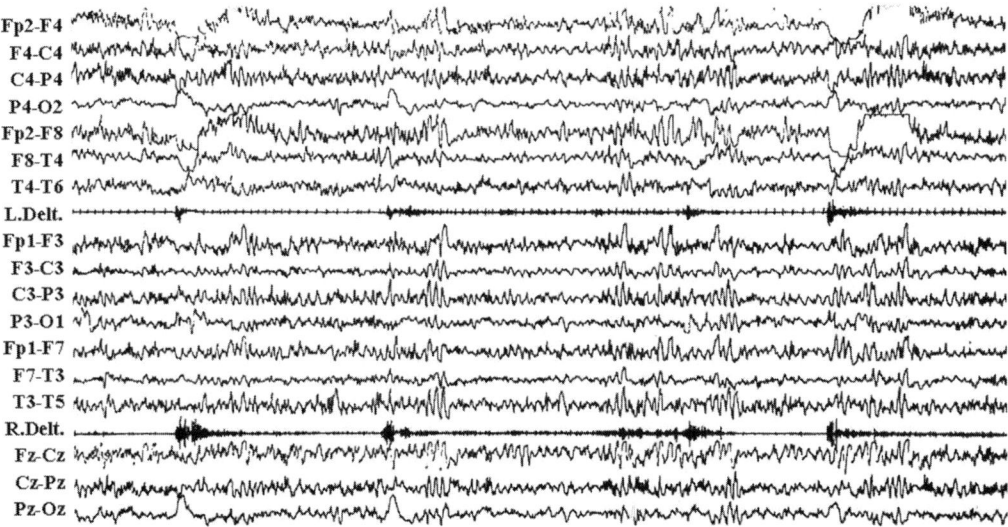

Figure 4. Infantile spasms in lissencephaly.
a. CT scan of the brain in a 14 months old girl with Miller-Dieker syndrome. There is a simplified gyral pattern with generalized pachygyria and ventricular dilatation.
b. The EEG during a series of spasms shows rhythmic background activity with high amplitude theta bursts, but no changes of electrogenesis are detectable during spasms, which are visible as bursts of diamond shaped EMG activity on both deltoids. (L. Delt = Left deltoid; R. Delt = right deltoid).

A
L. Delt
R. Scm
Fz-Cz
Cz-Pz
1 sec
100µV

B

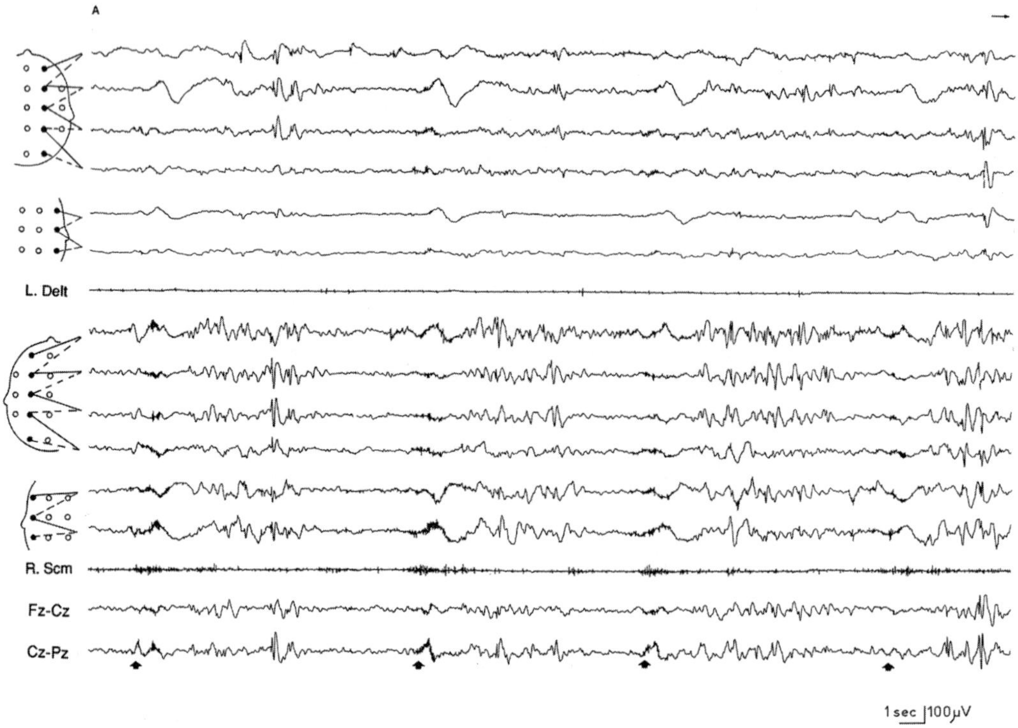

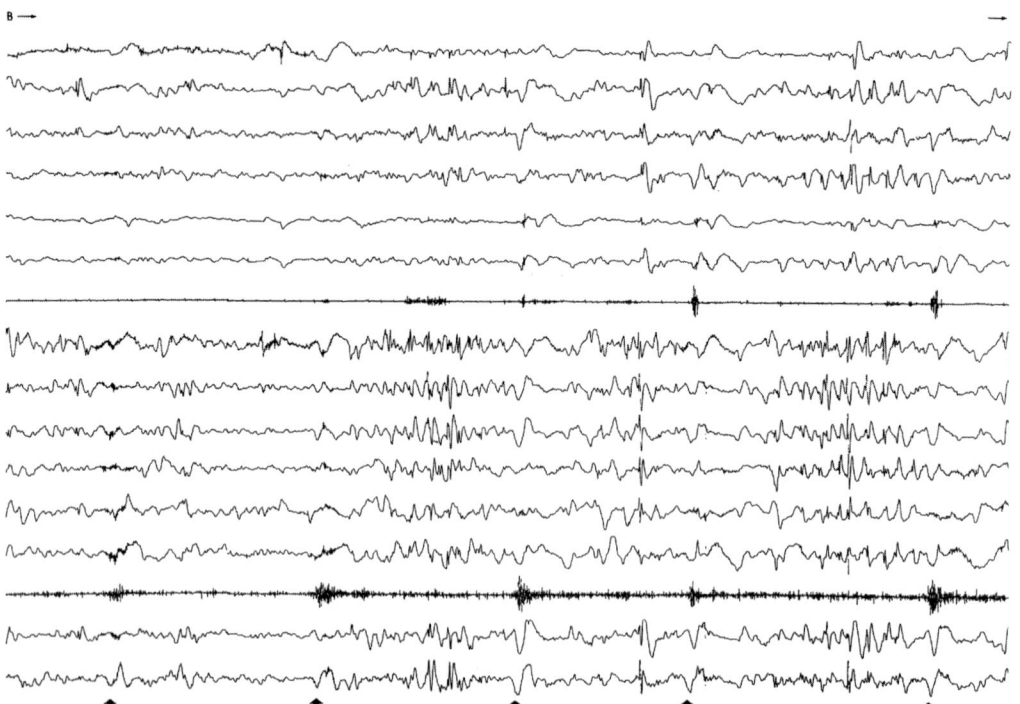

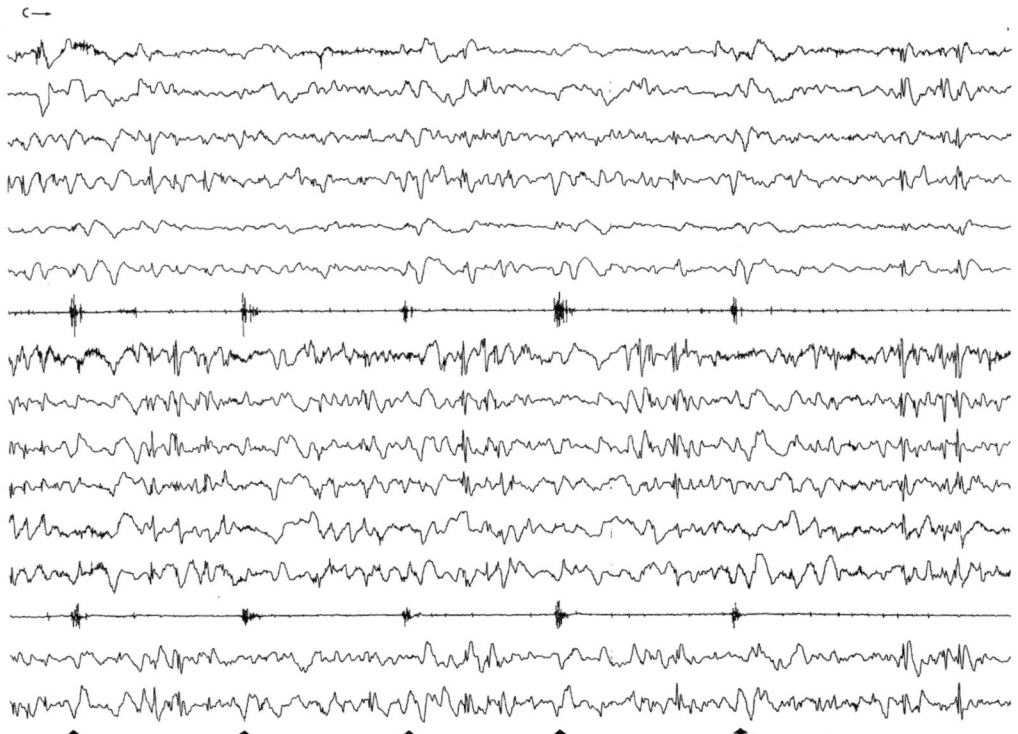

Figure 5. Asymmetric late onset spasms in a 8 year old boy with normal cognitive development.
a. Repetitive electrodecremental events (arrows) appear on the left hemisphere at the onset of a series of tonic spasms. Each event is separated by the next by irregular spike and wave activity and is accompanied on the EMG by a tonic contraction which is visible on the right sternocleidomastoideus muscle (R. Scm) while no EMG activity is recorded on the left (L. Delt = Left deltoid).
b. Tonic spasms become progressively more intense, and bilateral, acquiring a diamond shaped EMG morphology.
c. Spasms are bilateral and symmetric while EEG activity is progressively slower on the left hemisphere and electrodecremental event are less conspicuous.

Carbohydrate-deficient glycoprotein disorders and abnormalities of serine metabolism are rare but important causes as they are in part treatable. Pyridoxine dependency can rarely be first manifested by infantile spasms (Bankier et al., 1983; Krishnamoorthy, 1983), and this justifies a systematic trial of vitamin B_6.

West's syndrome results from acquired brain disorders in 8 to 14% of the cases (Arzimanoglou et al., 2004). Many causes of diffuse brain damage, whether inflammatory (herpes simplex), traumatic (subdural hematomas), anoxic, or ischemic, and, rarely, tumors have been associated to the syndrome (Asanuma et al., 1995; Arzimanoglou et al., 2004). Some reports have implicated immunization as an etiologic factor, the pertussis component usually being incriminated (Bellman et al., 1983). However, the association between infantile spasms and immunization is likely coincidental as the onset of spasms is often at an age when infants are normally vaccinated.

Clinical presentation *versus* etiology

The question as to whether discrete clinical pictures of infantile spasms are produced by different etiologic subgroups remains controversial. Some of the causes are associated with relatively specific clinical and EEG patterns, the most obvious examples being Aicardi's syndrome, hemimegalencephaly and, to a lesser extent, the lissencephaly spectrum of malformations and some cases of tuberous sclerosis (Paladin et al., 1989; Dalla Bernardina and Watanabe, 1994). Suggestive electroclinical features of idiopathic spasms have been proposed, as summarized above. However, there is no firm evidence suggesting that a subgroup exists with definite characteristics.

It has been suggested that IS might be a peculiar type of age related secondarily generalized seizures that can be triggered by focal paroxysmal activity arising from limited or more diffuse areas of abnormal cortex (Asano et al., 2001). Results of epilepsy surgery provide unquestionable support to the view that the abnormal cortex plays a key role in the initiation of seizures. Ictal FDG PET studies of infantile spasms have shown that hypometabolism involves focal cortical areas, as well as the lenticular nuclei and brainstem (Chugani et al., 1987; Juhasz et al., 2001), which might be in keeping with an interaction between such cortical and subcortical structures during spasms.

Late onset epileptic spasms

Gobbi et al. (1987) described as "periodic spasms" the clinical and EEG features in a series of children with severe encephalopathies. The typical presentation included a frequent onset by a focal seizure or EEG discharge, followed by a series of spasms, often asymmetrical or unilateral, each marked on the EEG by a slow complex with superimposed, low-amplitude, fast rhythms, without resumption of interictal activity between individual spasms. This electroclinical pattern has been repeatedly confirmed (Donat and Wright, 1991; Guerrini et al., 1992; Pachatz et al., 2003), even in adults (Cerullo et al., 1999) and appears to be the expression of developmental brain abnormalities. In older children and adults the epileptic spasms are the only manifestation that is reminiscent of the syndrome of infantile spasms, the clinical context being very different. Late onset spasms are almost invariably resistant to treatment. Although the outcome is usually regarded as poor, a number of cases are not associated with mental retardation or neurologic abnormalities *(Figure 5)*. In general, the later the onset of spasms the less the cognitive prognosis is influenced.

■ Prognosis in relation to etiology, imaging and EEG

The prognosis of infantile spasms is heavily influenced by the pathological process underlying the syndrome. Brain MRI has a high prognostic value, which is closely linked to its diagnostic power. Infants with normal MRI have the best prognosis (Saltik et al., 2002; Methahonkala et al., 2002). However, MRI may be normal in some metabolic disorders or dysplastic lesions that carry a poor prognosis.

Interictal FDG PET in children with infantile spasms and normal MRI, may show multifocal or diffuse hypometabolic patterns that may correlate with developmental outcome (Chugani et al., 1996). For example, bilateral hypometabolism in the temporal lobes correlated with an autistic disorder and a poor long term outcome (Chugani et al., 1996).

The prognostic value of the initial EEG characteristics is uncertain. Unilateral and grossly asymmetric tracings predict an unfavorable outcome, whereas a typical hypsarrhythmic pattern may be associated with a more favorable prognosis (Saltik et al., 2002). However, there is a limitation in the way studies on the prognostic value of EEG findings have been conducted. Prognosis of spasms and overall developmental prognosis have not been necessarily considered together. Experience with infants with large brain malformations suggests that hypsarrhythmia is often absent and that spasms persist well beyond the typical age range. This observation suggests that the typical hypsarrhythmic pattern requires at least some degree of anatomic and functional integrity of the brain in order to be generated. In addition, it seems that extensive brain malformations determine a sort of archaic or immature functional state where by only spasms or focal seizure can be generated even at an older age. It is therefore not surprising that prognosis for children exhibiting brain malformations and no typical hypsarrhythmia be guarded.

References

Archer HL, Evans J, Edwards S, Colley J, Newbury-Ecob R, O'Callaghan F, et al. CDKL5 mutations cause infantile spasms, early onset seizures, and severe mental retardation in female patients. *J Med Genet* 2006; 43: 729-34.

Arzimanoglou A, Guerrini R, Aicardi J. Aicardi's Epilepsy in Children. Third edition. Philadelphia: Lippincott Williams & Williams, 2004, 516 p.

Asano E, Chugani DC, Juhasz C, Muzik O, Chugani HT. Surgical treatment of West syndrome. *Brain Dev* 2001; 23: 668-76.

Asanuma H, Wakai S, Tanaka T, Chiba S. Brain tumors associated with infantile spasms. *Pediatr Neurol* 1995; 12: 361-4.

Bankier A, Turner M, Hopkins IJ. Pyridoxine dependent seizures – a wider clinical spectrum. *Arch Dis Childh* 1983; 58: 415-8.

Barkovich AJ, Kuzniecky RI, Jackson GD, Guerrini R, Dobyns WB. A developmental and genetic classification for malformation of cortical development. *Neurology* 2005; 65: 1873-87.

Barkovich AJ, Guerrini R, Battaglia G, Kalifa G, N'Guyen T, Parmeggiani A, et al. Band heterotopia: correlation of outcome with magnetic resonance imaging parameters. *Ann Neurol* 1994; 36: 609-17.

Bastos AC, Comeau RM, Andermann F, Melanson D, Cendes F, Dubeau F, et al. Diagnosis of subtle focal dysplastic lesions: curvilinear reformatting from three-dimensional magnetic resonance imaging. *Ann Neurol* 1999; 46: 88-94.

Bednarek N, Motte J, Soufflet C, Plouin P, Dulac O. Evidence of late-onset infantile spasms. *Epilepsia* 1998; 39: 55-60.

Bellman MH, Ross EM, Miller DL. Infantile spasms and pertussis immunisation. *Lancet* 1983; 1: 1031-4.

Cao A, Cianchetti C, Signorini E, Loi M, Sanna G, De Vergilis S. Agenesis of the corpus callosum, infantile spasms, spastic quadriplegia, microcephaly and severe mental retardation in three siblings. *Clin Genet* 1977; 12: 290-6.

Caplan C, Guthrie D, Mundy P, Sigman M, Shiels D, Sherman T, Peacock WJ. Non-verbal communication skills of surgically treated children with infantile spasms. *Dev Med Child Neurol* 1992; 34: 499-506.

Carbonara C, Longa L, Grosso E, Borrone C, Garre MG, Brisigotti M, et al. 9q34 loss of heterozygosity in a tuberous sclerosis astrocytoma suggests a growth suppressor-like activity also for the TSC1 gene. *Hum Molec Genet* 1994; 3: 1829-1832.

Cerullo A, Marini C, Carcangiu R, Baruzzi A, Tinuper P. Clinical and video-polygraphic features of epileptic spasms in adults with cortical migration disorder. *Epileptic Disord* 1999; 1: 27-33.

Chan S, Chin SS, Nordli DR, Goodman RR, DeLaPaz RL, Pedley TA. Prospective magnetic resonance imaging identification of focal cortical dysplasia, including the non-balloon cell subtype. *Ann Neurol* 1998; 44: 749-57.

Chevrie JJ, Aicardi J. Le pronostic psychique des spasmes infantiies traités par l'ACTH ou les corticoïdes. Analyse statistique de 78 cas suivis plus d'un an. *J Neurol Sci* 1971; 12: 351-7.

Chevrie JJ, Aicardi J. Convulsive disorders in the first year of life. Etiologic factors. *Epilepsia* 1977; 18: 489-98.

Chevrie JJ. Aicardi J, The Aicardi syndrome. In: Pedley TA, Meldrum BS, eds. *Recent advances in Epilepsy vol. 3*. Edinburgh: Churchill Livingstone, 1986: 189-210.

Chugani HT, Da Silva E, Chugani DC. Infantile spasms: III. Prognostic implications of bitemporal hypometabolism on positron emission tomography. *Annals of Neurology* 1996; 39: 643-9.

Chugani HT, Mazziota JC, Ergel J Jr, Phelps ME. The Lennox-Gastaut syndrome: Metabolic subtypes determined by 2-Dioxy-2 ^{18}F fluoro-D-glucose positron emission tomography. *Ann. Neurol* 1987; 21: 4-13.

Ciardo F, Zamponi N, Specchio N, Parmeggiani L, Guerrini R. Autosomal recessive polymicrogyria with infantile spasms and limb deformities. *Neuropediatrics* 2001; 32: 325-9.

Claes S, Devriendt K, Lagae L, Ceulemans B, Dom L, Casaer P, Raeymaekers P, Cassiman JJ, Fryns JP. The X-linked infantile spasms syndrome (MIM 308350) maps to Xp11.4-Xpter in two pedigrees. *Ann Neurol* 1997; 42: 360-4.

Coleman M, Hart PN, Randall J, Lee J, Hijada D, Bratenahl CG. Serotonin levels in the blood and central nervous system of a patient with sudanophilic leukodystrophy. *NeuroPédiatrie* 1977; 8: 459-66.

Curatolo P. Tuberous sclerosis: relationships between clinical and EEG findings and magnetic resonance imaging. In: Guerrini R, Andermann F, Canapicchi R, Roger J, Zifkin B, Pfanner P, eds. *Dysplasias of cerebral cortex and epilepsy*. Philadelphia: Lippincott-Raven, 1996: 191-8.

Curatolo P, Seri S, Verdecchia M, Bombardieri R. Infantile spasms in tuberous scleroris complex. *Brain Dev* 2001; 23: 502-7.

Coulter D L. Continuous infantile spasms as a form of status epilepticus. *J Child Neurol* 1986; 1: 215-7.

Dabora SL, Jozwiak S, Franz DN, Roberts PS, Nicto A, Chung J, *et al*. Mutational analysis in a cohort of 224 tuberous sclerosis patients indicates increased severity of TSC2, compared with TSC1, disease in multiple organs. *Am J Hum Genet* 2001; 68: 64-80.

Dalla Bernardina B, Watanabe K. Interictal EEG: variations and pitfalls. In: Dulac O, Chugani HT, Dalla Bernardina B, eds. *Infantile Spasms and West Syndrome*. Philadelphia: WB Saunders, 1994: 63-81.

de Menezes MA, Rho JM. Clinical and electrographic features of epileptic spasms persisting beyond the second year of life. *Epilepsia* 2002; 43: 623-30.

Dobyns WB, Berry-Kravis E, Havernick NJ, Holden KR, Viskochil D. X-linked lissencephaly with absent corpus callosum and ambiguous genitalia. *Am J Med Genet* 1999; 86: 331-7.

Dravet C, Giraud N, Bureau M, Roger J, Gobbi G, Dalla Bernardina B. Benign myoclonus of early infancy or benign non-epileptic spasms. *Neuropediatrics* 1986; 17: 33-8.

Donat JF, Wright FS. Simultaneous infantile spasms and partial seizures. *J Child Neurol* 1991; 6: 246-50.

Dulac O. Infantile spasms and West syndrome. In: Engel JJr and Pedley T eds. *Epilepsy: a comprehensive textbook*. Philadelphia: Lippincott-Raven, 1997: 2277-83.

Dulac O. What is West syndrome? *Brain Dev* 2001; 23: 447-52.

Dulac O, Chugani T, Dalla Bernardina B. Overview. In: Dulac O, Chugani T, Dalla Bernardina B. eds. *Infantile spasms and West sindrome*. London: Saunders, 1994: 1-5.

Dulac O, Pinard JM, Plouin P. Infantile spasms associated with cortical dysplasia and tuberous sclerosis. In: Guerrini R, Andermann F, Canapicchi R, eds. *Dysplasias of Cerebral Cortex and Epilepsy*. Philadelphia: Lippincott-Raven, 1996: 217-25.

Dulac O, Plouin P, Jambaqué I, and Motte J. Spasmes infantiles épileptiques bénins. *Rev EEG Neurophysiol Clin* 1986; 16: 371-82.

Dulac O, Plouin P, Perulli L, Diebler C, Arthuis M, Jalin C. Aspects électroencéphalographiques de l'agyrie-pachygyrie classique. *Rev. EEG Neurophysiol Clin* 1983; 13: 232-9.

Egli M, Mothersill I, O'Kane M, O'Kane F. The axial spasm – The predominant type of drop seizure in patients with secondary generalized epilepsy. *Epilepsia* 1985; 26: 401-15.

Eriksson SH, Rugg-Gunn FJ, Symms MR, Barker GJ, Duncan JS. Diffusion tensor imaging in patients with epilepsy and malformation of cortical development. *Brain* 2001; 124: 617-26.

European Chromosome 16 Tuberous Sclerosis Consortium. Identification and characterization of the tuberous sclerosis on chromosome 16. *Cell* 1993; 75: 1305-15.

Fejerman N, Caraballo R. Appendix to Shuddering and benign myoclonus of early infancy. In. *Epilepsy and movement disorders*. R. Guerrini, J. Aicardi, F. Andermann, M. Hallett eds. Cambridge: University Press, 2002: 349-51.

Fleiszar KA, Daniel WL, Imrey PB. Genetic study of infantile spasms with hypsarrhythmia. *Epilepsia* 1977; 18: 55-62.

Fusco L, Vigevano F. Ictal clinical electroencephalographic findings of spasms in West syndrome. *Epilepsia* 1993; 34: 671-8.

Fusco L, Pachatz C, Cusmai R, Vigevano F. Repetitive sleep starts in neurologically impaired children: an unusual non-epileptic manifestation in otherwise epileptic subjects. *Epileptic Disord* 1999; 1: 63-7.

Gaily E, Liukkonen E, Paetau R, Rekola R, Granstrom ML. Infantile spasms: diagnosis and assessment of treatment response by video-EEG. *Dev Med Child Neurol* 2001; 43: 658-67.

Gastaut H, Pinsard N, Raybaud C, Aicardi J, Zifkin B. Lissencephaly (agyria-pachygyria): clinical findings and serial EEG studies. *Dev Med Child Neurol* 1987; 29: 167-80.

Gobbi G, Bruno L, Pini A, Rossi PG, Tassinari CA. Periodic spasms: An unclassified type of epileptic seizure in childhood. *Dev Med Child Neurol* 1987; 27: 766-75.

Guerrini R. Epilepsy in children. *Lancet* 2006; 367: 499-524.

Guerrini R, Carrozzo R. Epilepsy and genetic malformations of the cerebral cortex. *Am J Med Genet* 2001a; 106: 160-73.

Guerrini R, Carrozzo R. Epileptogenic brain malformations: clinical presentation, malformative patterns and indications for genetic testing. *Seizure* 2001b; 10: 532-47.

Guerrini R, Marini C. Genetic malformations of cortical development. *Exp Brain Res* 2006; 173 (2): 322-33.

Guerrini R, Belmonte A, Carrozzo R. Paroxysmal tonic upgaze of childhood with ataxia: a benign transient dystonia with autosomal dominant inheritance. *Brain Dev* 1998; 20: 116-8.

Guerrini R, Andermann E, Avoli M, Dobyns WB. Cortical dysplasias, genetics and epileptogenesis. *Adv Neurol* 1999; 79: 95-121.

Guerrini R, Robain O, Dravet C, Canapicchi R, Roger J. Clinical, electrographic and pathological findings in the gyral disorders. In: Fejerman N, Chamoles NA, eds. *New trends in pediatric neurology*. Amsterdam: Elsevier, 1993: 101-7.

Guerrini R, Andermann F, Canapicchi R, Roger J, Zifkin BG, Pfanner P, eds. *Dysplasias of cerebral cortex and epilepsy*. Philadephia: Lippincott-Raven, 1996, 461 p.

Guerrini R, Genton P, Dravet C, Viallat D, Bureau M, Horton EJ, et al. Compulsive somatosensory self stimulation inducing epileptic seizures. *Epilepsia* 1992; 33: 509-16.

Haga Y, Watanabe K, Negoro T, Aso K, Kasai K, Ohki T, Natume J. Do ictal, clinical, and electroencephalographic features predict outcome in West syndrome? *Pediatr Neurol* 1995; 13: 226-9.

Hrachovy RA, and Frost JD. Infantile spasms. *Pediatric Clinics of North America* 1989; 36: 311-30.

Hrachovy RA, Frost JD, Kellaway P. Hypsarrhythmia, variations on the theme. *Epilepsia* 1984; 25: 317-25.

Ikeno T, Shigematsu H, Miyakushi M, Ohba A, Yagi K, Seino M. An analytic study of epileptic falls. *Epilepsia* 1985; 26: 612-21.

Jambaqué I, Cusmai R, Curatolo P, Cortesi F, Perrot C, Dulac O. Neuropsychological aspects of Tuberous Sclerosis in relation to epilepsy and MRI findings. *Dev Med Child Neurol* 1991; 33: 698-705.

Jambaqué I, Chiron C, Dulac O, Raynaud C, Syrota P. Visual inattention in West syndrome: a neuropsychological and neurofunctional imaging study. *Epilepsia* 1993; 34: 692-700.

Juhasz C, Chugani HT, Muzik O, Chugani DC. Neuroradiological assessment of brain structure and function and its implication in the pathogenesis of West syndrome. *Brain Dev* 2001; 23: 488-95.

Kato M, Das S, Petras K, Sawaishi Y, Dobyns WB. Polyalanine expansion of ARX associated with cryptogenic West syndrome. *Neurology* 2003; 61: 267-76.

Kato M, Das S, Petras K, et al. Mutations of ARX are associated with striking pleiotropy and consistent genotype-phenotype correlation. *Hum Mutat* 2004; 23: 147-59.

Kellaway P, Frost JD, Hrachovy RA. Infantile spasms. In: Morselli PL, Pippenger CE, Penry JK, eds. *Antiepileptic Drug Therapy*. New York: Raven Press, 1983: 115-36.

Kellaway P, Hrachovy RA, Frost JD, Zion T. Precise characterization and quantification of infantile spasms. *Ann Neurol* 1979; 6: 214-8.

King M, Stephenson JBP, Ziervogel M, Doyle D, Galbraith S. Hemimegalencephaly – A case for hemispherectomy. *Neuropediatrics* 1985; 16: 46-55.

Koo B, Hwang P. Localization of focal cortical lesions influences age of onset of infantile spasms. *Epilepsia* 1996; 37: 1068-71.

Krishnamoorthy KS. Pyridoxine-dependency seizure: Report of a rare presentation. *Ann Neurol* 1983; 13: 103-4.

Lacy JR, Penry JK. *Infantile Spasms*. New York 1976: Raven Press.

Lombroso CT. A prospective study of infantile spasms: Clinical and therapeutic correlations. *Epilepsia* 1983; 24: 135-58.

Mari F, Azimonti S, Bertani I, Bolognese F, Colombo E, Caselli R, et al. CDKL5 belongs to the same molecolar pathway of MeCP2 and it is responsible for the early-onset seizure variant of Rett syndrome. *Human Molecular Genetics* 2005; 14 (14): 1935-46.

Methahonkala L, Gaily E, Rantala H, Salmi E, Valanne L, Aarimaa T, et al. Focal and global cortical hypometabolism in patients with newly diagnosed infantile spasms. *Neurology* 2002; 58: 1646-51.

Motte J, Billard C, Fejerman N, Sfaello Z, Arroyo H, Dulac O. Neurofibromatosis type one and West syndrome: a relatively benign association. *Epilepsia* 1993; 34: 723-6.

Nabbout R, Melki I, Gerbaka B, Dulac O, Akatcherian C. Infantile spasms in Down syndrome: good response to a short course of vigabatrin. *Epilepsia* 2001; 42: 1580-3.

Paladin F, Chiron C, Dulac O, Plouin P, Ponsot G. Electroencephalographic aspects of hemimegalencephaly. *Dev Med Child Neurol* 1989; 31: 377-83.

Pachatz C, Fusco L, Vigevano F. Epileptic spasms and partial seizures as a single ictal event. *Epilepsia* 2003; 44: 693-700.

Plouin P, Jalin C, Dulac O, Chiron C. Enregistrement ambulatoire de l'EEG pendant 24 heures dans les spasmes infantiles épileptiques. *Rev EEG Neurophysiol Clin* 1987; 17: 309-18.

Poley JR, Dumermuth G. EEG findings in patients with phenylketonuria before and during treatment with a low phenylalanine diet and in patients with some other inborn errors of metabolism. In: Holt KS, Coffey VP, eds. *Some Recent Advances in Inborn Errors of Metabolism*, Edinburgh: Churchill-Livingstone, 1968: 61-9.

Quirk JA, Kendall B, Kingsley DP, Boyd SG, Pitt MC. EEG features of cortical dysplasia in children. *Neuropediatrics* 1993; 24 (4): 193-9.

Reiter E, Tiefenthaler M, Freillinger M, Bernert G, Seidl R, Hauser E. Familial idiopathic West syndrome. *J Child Neurol* 2000; 15: 249-52.

Riikonen R. Infantile spasms: Modem practical aspects. *Act. Paediatr Scand* 1984; 73: 1-6.

Riikonen R. Epidemiological data of West syndrome in Finland. *Brain Dev* 2001; 23: 539-41.

Robain O, Vinters HV Neuropathologic studies. In: Dulac O, Chugani HT, Dalla Bernardina B, eds. *Infantile Spasms and West Syndrome*. Philadelphia: W.B. Saunders, 1994: 99-117.

Roger J, Dravet Ch, Boniver C, et al. L'épilepsie dans la Sclérose Tubéreuse de Bourneville. *Boll Lega It Epil* 1984; 45/46: 33-8.

Saltik S, Kocer N, Dervent A. Informative value of magnetic resonance imaging and EEG in the prognosis of infantile spasms. *Epilepsia* 2002; 43: 246-52.

Sankar R, Curran JG, Kevill JW, Rintahaka PJ, Shewmon DA, Vinters HV. Microscopic cortical dysplasia in infantile spasms: evolution of white matter abnormalities. *AJNR Am J Neuroradiol* 1995; 16: 1265-72.

Scala E, Ariani F, Mari F, Caselli R, Pescucci C, Longo I, et al. CDKL5/STK9 is mutated in Rett sindrome variant with infantile spasms. *J Med Genet* 2005; 42: 103-7.

Silva ML, Cieuta C, Guerrini R, Plouin P, Livet MO, Dulac O. Early clinical and EEG features of infantile spasms in Down syndrome. *Epilepsia* 1996; 37: 977-82.

Stafstrom CE, Konkol RJ. Infantile spasms in children with Down syndrome. *Dev Med Chil Neurol* 1994; 36: 576-85.

Stafstrom CE, Patxot CE, Gilmore HE, Wisniewski KE. Seizures in children with Down syndrome: etiology, characteristics and outcome. *Dev Med Child Neurol* 1991; 33: 191-200.

Stromme P, Sundet K, Mork C, Cassiman JJ, Fryns JP, Claes S. X linked mental retardation and infantile spasms in a family: new clinical data and linkage to Xp11.4-Xp22.11. *J Med Genet* 1999; 36: 374-8.

Stromme P, Mangelsdorf ME, Shaw MA, Lower KM, Lewis SM, Bruyere H, et al. Mutations in the human ortholog of Aristaless cause X-linked mental retardation and epilepsy. *Nat Genet* 2002; 30: 441-5.

Sugai K, Fukuyama Y, Yasuda K, Fujimoto S, Ohtsu M, Ohta H, et al. Clinical and pedigree study on familial cases of West syndrome in Japan. *Brain Dev* 2001; 123: 558-64.

Van Slegtenhorst M, de Hoogt R, Hermans C, Nellist M, Janssen B, Verhoef S, et al. Identification of the tuberous sclerosis gene TSC1 on chromosome 9q34. *Science* 1997; 277: 805-8.

Vigevano F, Di Rocco C. Effectiveness of hemispherectomy in hemimegalencephaly with intractable seizures. *Neuropediatrics* 1990; 21: 222-3.

Vigevano F, Fusco L, Pachatz C. Related Articles Neurophysiology of spasms. *Brain Dev* 2001; 23: 467-72.

Vigevano F, Fusco L, Cusmai R, Claps D, Ricci S, Dilani L. The idiopathic form of West syndrome. *Epilepsia* 1993; 34: 743-6.

Weaving LS, Christodoulou J, Williamson SL, Friend KL, McKenzie OLD, Archer H, et al. Mutation of CDKL5 Cause e Severe Neurodevelopmental Disorder with Infantile Spasms and Mental Retardation. *Am J Hum Genet* 2004; 75: 1079-93.

Yamamoto N, Watanabe K, Negoro T. Partial seizures evolving to infantile spasms. *Epilepsia* 1988; 29: 34-40.

Epileptic spasms: interictal patterns

Bernardo Dalla Bernardina, Elena Fontana, Elisa Osanni,
Roberta Opri, Francesca Darra

Child Neuropsychiatry Unit, University of Verona, Italy

Defining or even only describing the interictal patterns of West syndrome is a very difficult task because of the ambiguity concerning the definitions of West syndrome and of the boundaries between ictal and interictal EEG.

West syndrome, according to the most recent West Delphi group Consensus (Lux and Osborne 2004) is considered a subset of infantile spasms, characterized by the association of infantile spasms and hypsarrhythmia. Nevertheless the same West Delphi group concludes that consensus was not reached on how to define EEG criteria and hypsarrhythmia.

The term "hypsarrhythmia" was coined by Gibbs and Gibbs (1952) for identifying the interictal patterns commonly associated with infantile spasms and was described as follows: "... random high voltage slow waves and spikes. These spikes vary from moment to moment, both in duration and location. At times they appear to be focal, and a few seconds later they seem to originate from multiple foci. Occasionally, the spike discharge becomes generalized, but it never appears as a rhythmically repetitive and highly organized pattern that could be confused with a discharge of the petit mal variant type. The abnormality is almost continuous, and in most cases it shows as clearly in the waking as in the sleeping record. It is referred to as hypsarrhythmia."

The West Delphi group definition is substantially analogous (Lux and Osborne, 2004): "... an EEG pattern that is characterised by random, high-voltage spikes and slow waves. The most striking features of hypsarrhythmia are high-voltage (generally > 200 µV) slow waves with variable amplitude; spikes and waves from many foci, and varying with time; and a lack of synchrony, with a generally "chaotic" appearance."

The "multifocality" that is easily highlighted by modifying the recording parameters (by excluding slow waves from EEG using a digital filter) *(Figure 1)*, as well documented by Oka *et al.* (2004), in some cases can simply reflect the cerebral maturation process of infancy (Chiron *et al.*, 1992; Dulac, 2001; Guzzetta *et al.*, 2002; Oka *et al.*, 2004) *(Figure 1)*, while in others it is related to a focal cortical lesion (Ohtsuka

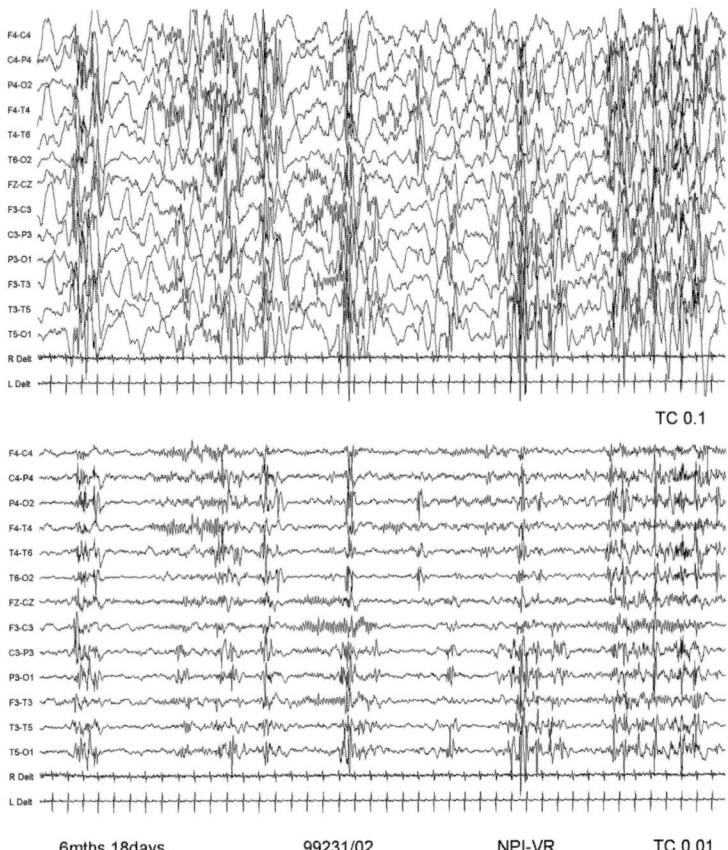

Figure 1. Six months 18 days old girl with normal development showing from 16 days infantile spasms in clusters, impairment of visual contact and typical hypsarrhythmia while awake. Brain MRI is normal. By excluding slow waves (bottom) (TC 0.01) it is possible to enhance the evidence of multifocal spikes difficult to recognize with routing recording (TC 0.1) (top). Diffuse and focal paroxysms and IS disappear in a few days after ACTH therapy. At present she is 4 years old without treatment and developing normally; the EEG is normal both during wake and sleep.

et al., 1996; Suzuki et al., 2003). In these cases the focality is stable, correlates with an equally stable clinical pattern (*Figure 2*) and generally persists after hypsarrhythmia pattern resolution by therapy (*Figure 3*).

In the two definitions the common elements are the predominantly diffuse and almost continuous paroxysms with high amplitude, their chaotic organization, the apparent multifocality and the subcontinuous fluctuation of the whole picture.

This hypsarrhythmic pattern can be modified by vigilance. During drowsiness and non-REM sleep there is an increase of spikes and polispikes (Gastaut et al., 1964). In non-REM sleep it appears more fragmented (Kellaway et al., 1983), while during REM sleep it is strongly reduced (Hrachovy et al., 1981) (*Figure 4*). In some cryptogenic or symptomatic cases, the picture appears truly hypsarrhythmic only during drowsiness (*Figure 5*).

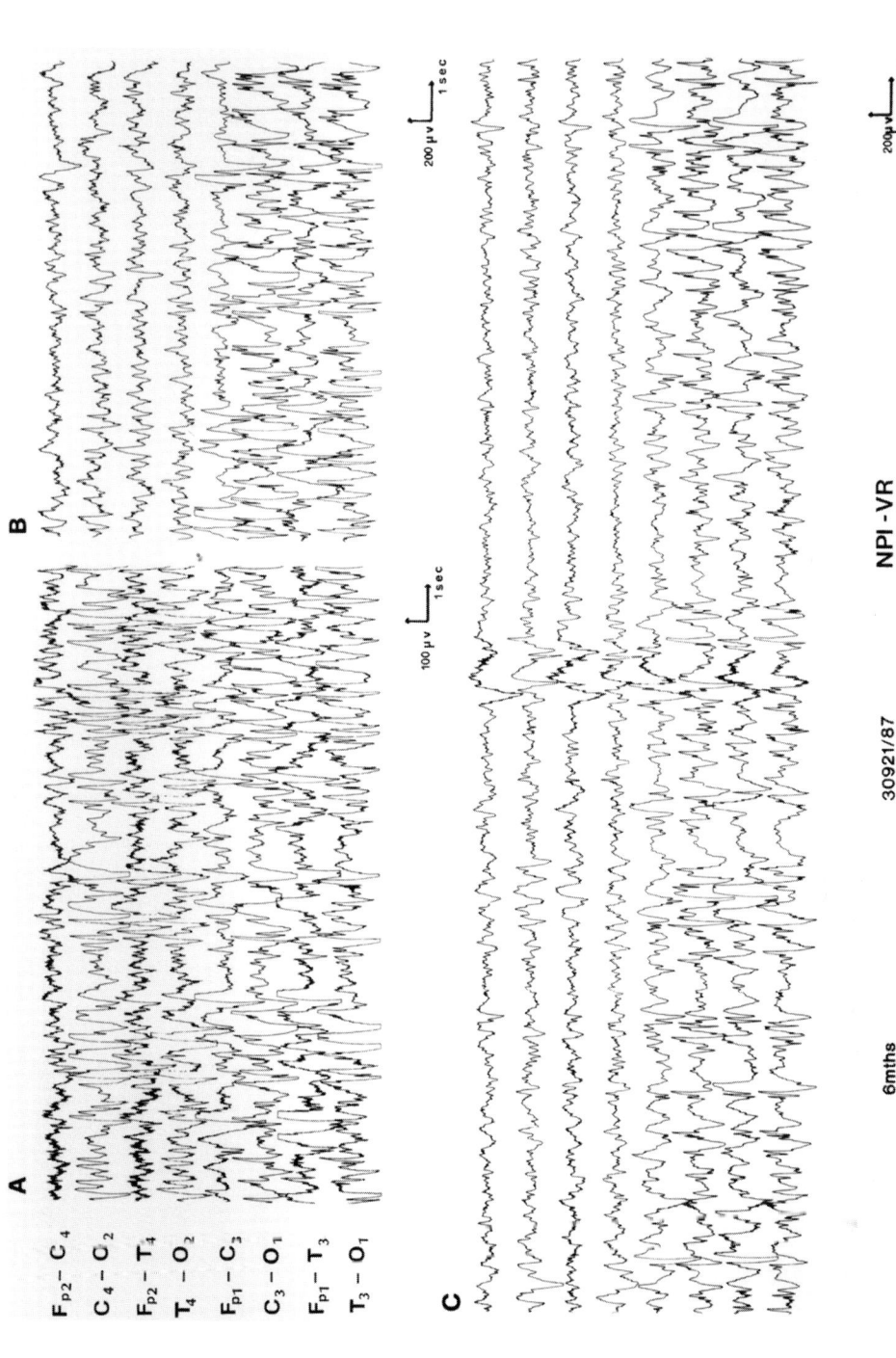

Figure 2. Six months old boy with a prenatal left occipital poroencephaly who presented infantile spasms in clusters since the age of 3 months 20 days.
(Upper right) By diminishing the amplitude it is possible to recognise the mainly unilateral expression of hypsarrhythmia persisting during the occurrence of bilateral spasms (below).

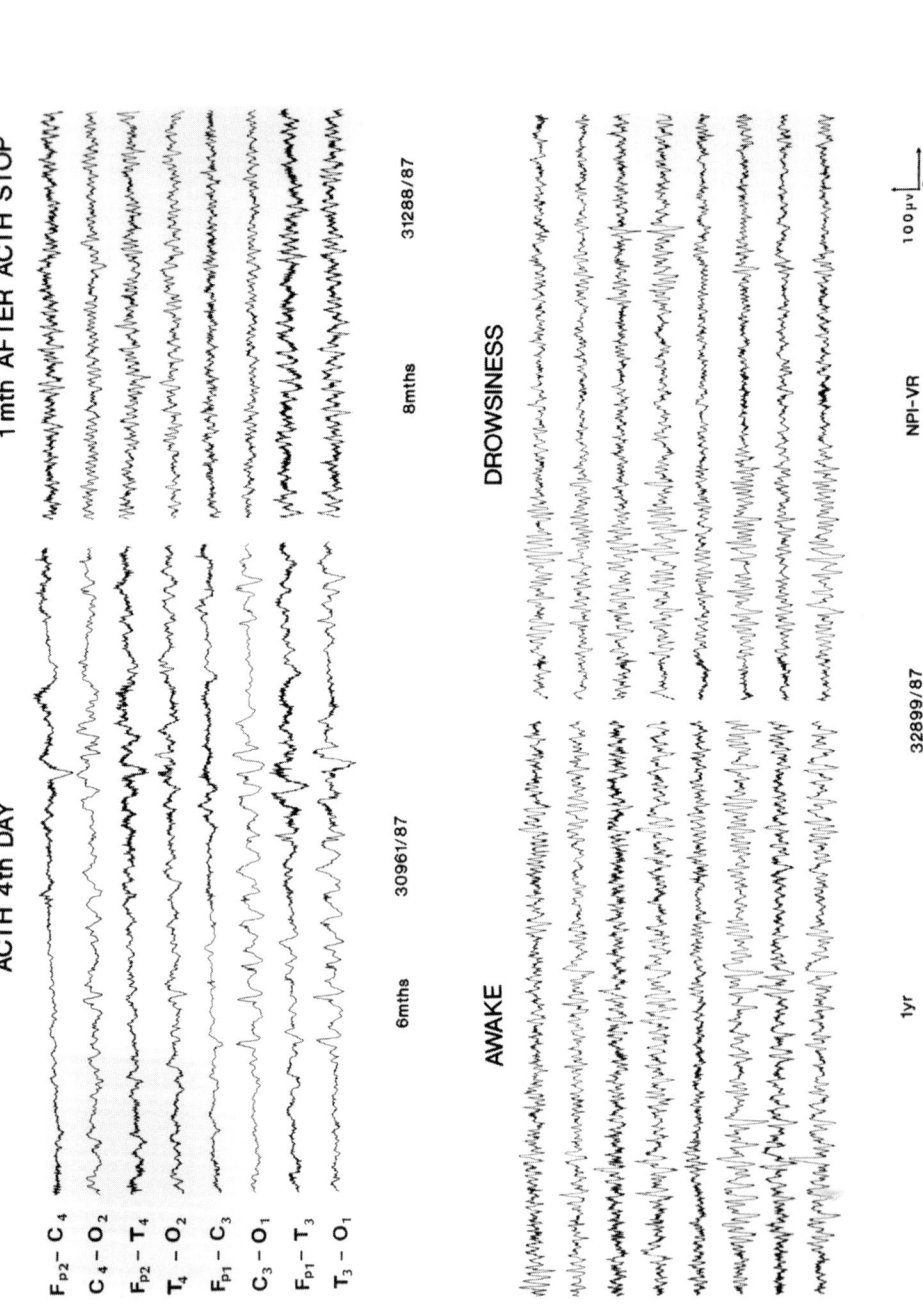

Figure 3. Same case as Figure 2.
With vanishing of hypsarrhythmia, we can easily recognize focal paroxysms involving the left occipital region persisting throughout evolution even after seizures and treatment stop. At the age of 5 years a typical picture of CSWS will appear with concomitant learning and behavioural problems well controlled by ethosuximide.

Epileptic spasms: interictal patterns

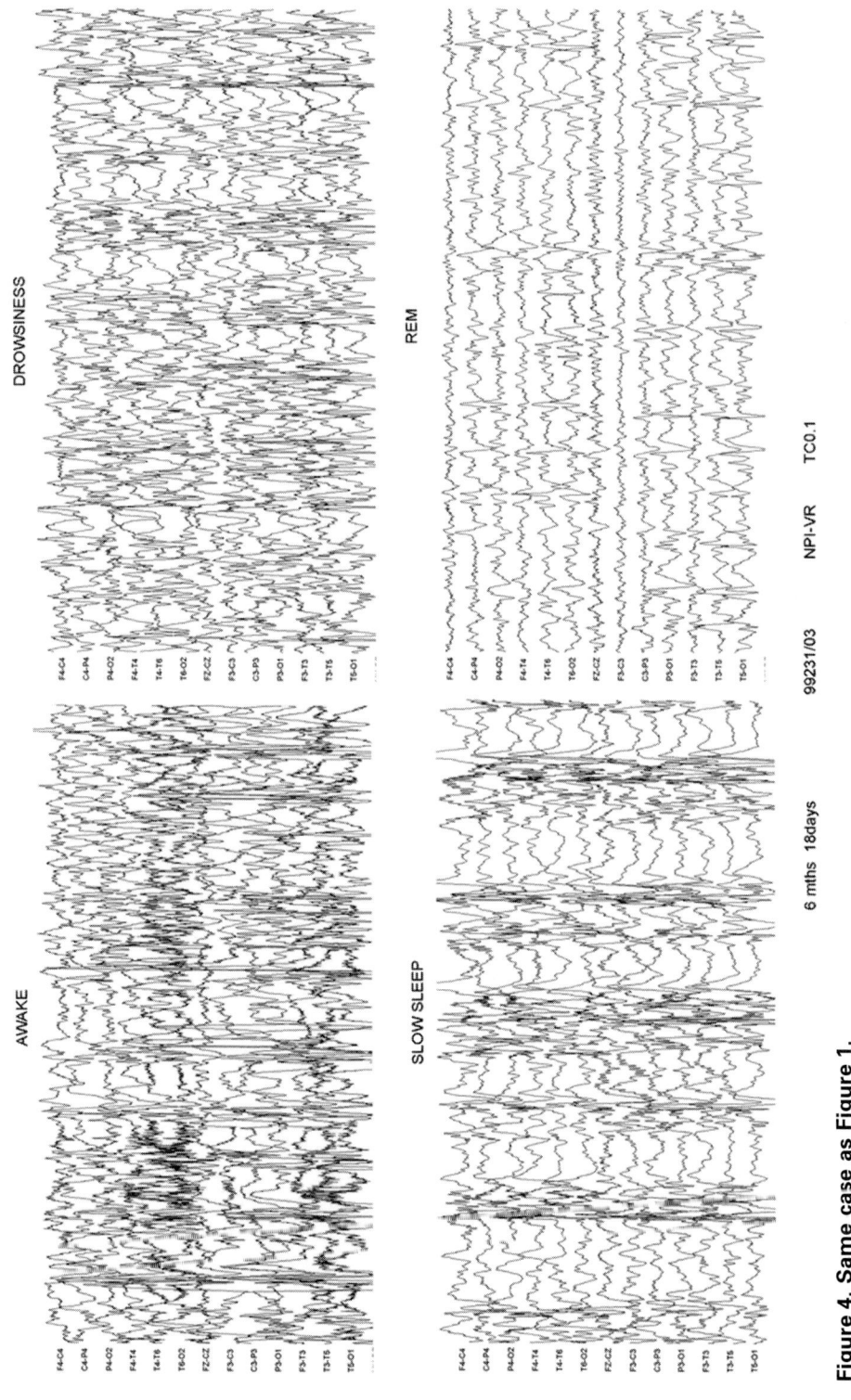

Figure 4. Same case as Figure 1.
The hypsarrhythmic pattern is reinforced during drowsiness, while it results more fragmented during slow sleep with easily recognizable spindles. During REM sleep the hypsarrhythmic pattern disappears while apparently multifocal paroxysms, mainly located posteriorly, persist. At present he is 19 years old and is studying at university level.

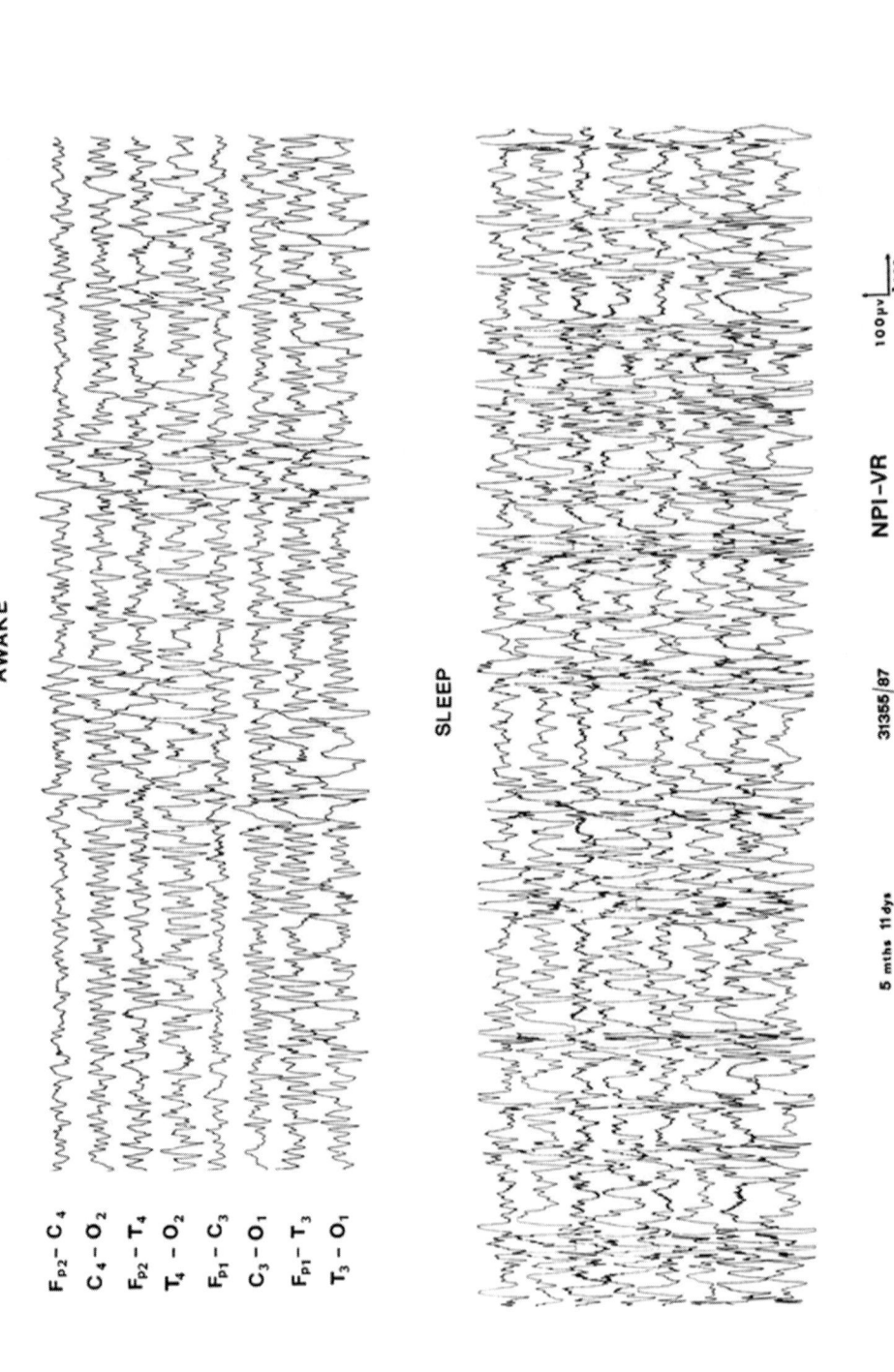

Figure 5. Five months old boy with normal development and normal brain CT scan, suffering since a few days from infantile spasms in clusters.
We can observe as the EEG pattern becomes truly hypsarrhythmic only during sleep. Following ACTH treatment infantile spasms disappeared with concomitant EEG normalization both during wake and sleep.

On the other hand it has been well documented that hypsarrhythmia can be modified by vigilance as well as additional factors such as type and topography of the underlying pathology, age, duration of disorder, frequency and manner of recurrence of ictal events, treatment and obviously other factors given by the many combinations of these. Hypsarrhythmia morphology can also be strongly conditioned by the coexistence of unusual EEG activities, like for example cases with cortical dysplasia (Dalla Bernardina et al., 1996). Evaluation of the picture also depends on recording parameters and duration.

According to these variables some Authors (Gastaut, 1970; Lombroso, 1983; Hrachovy et al., 1984; Hrachovy and Frost, 2003) described some modified or atypical pictures resulting in relatively well defined variants. The term atypical should be discarded because used by some Authors (Pachioli and Cavazzuti, 1962; Sorel, 1978) for identifying cases of atypical West Syndrome (spasms without hypsarrhythmia or hypsarrhythmia without spasms).

The unanimously recognized variants are the following:
- Hypsarrhythmia with increased inter-hemispheric synchronization, realizing at times a more fragmented picture while awake, in which the multifocal spike and sharp wave activity and the diffuse asynchronous slow wave activity are replaced or intermingled with activity that exhibits a significant degree of interhemispheric synchrony and symmetry.
- Asymmetric hypsarrhythmia also referred to as hemi-hypsarrhythmia or unilateral hypsarrhythmia characterized by hypsarrhythmia with a consistent difference in amplitude between hemispheres.
- Hypsarrhythmia with a consistent focus of abnormal discharges in which a distinct focus of spike or sharp wave activity is superimposed on a typical hypsarrhythmic background often tending to persist after disappearance of the hypsarrhythmic pattern.
- Hypsarrhythmia with episodes of voltage attenuation referred to as the suppression burst variant of hypsarrhythmia, characterized by a hypsarrhthmic pattern interrupted by episodes of generalized, regional or localized voltage attenuation, that typically persist from 2 to a few seconds.
- Hypsarrhythmia with high voltage slow activity with little or no spike/sharp wave components (excessive slowing) consisting of high-voltage, asynchronous and synchronous slow activity with little or no spike/sharp wave components.
- Hypsarrhythmia with predominant fast activity (excessive rapidity) consisting in a picture modified by the coexistence of fast activities or an increase of the fast poly-spikes component.

As recently recommended by the West Delphi group Consensus (Lux and Osborne, 2004) one should notice that many of these features are a matter of degree rather than absolute differences. According to these variants several Authors have attempted to make correlations to the nature of epilepsy and/or specific neuropathology. The probability of a symptomatic rather than cryptogenic aetiology seems to be higher in cases with a variant rather than typical hypsarrhythmia (Pachioli and Cavazzuti, 1962; Gastaut, 1970, Jeavons and Bower, 1974; Dulac et al., 1993; Fusco and

Vigevano, 1993; Dalla Bernardina and Watanabe; 1994; Dulac et al., 1994; Hrachovy and Frost, 2003; Dulac and Tuxhorn, 2005). This hypothesis appears reinforced if the interictal paroxysms disappear during the cluster of spasms and if there are associated partial seizures and/or persisting focal EEG paroxysms. In any case these patterns are highly influenced by the underlying pathology, the course of the disorder, treatment, vigilance status, age and semeiology and frequency of seizures and manner of recurrence.

Finally we must remember, that in many cases hypsarrhythmia has not been observed, (Druckman and Chao, 1955; Pachioli and Cavazzuti, 1962; Watanabe et al., 1973; Jeavons and Bower, 1974; Sorel, 1978; Watanabe et al., 1993; Dalla Bernardina and Watanabe, 1994; Ohtahara and Yamatogi, 2001), neither have any type of paroxysmal abnormalities (Caraballo et al., 2003).

Although the analysis, case by case, of the electroclinical picture can help diagnostic definition and prognostic evaluation, variants or modified patterns *per se* are frequent and generally not correlated to prognosis and only partially to aethiology (Kramer et al., 1997). So probably as already recommended by the Royaumont Workshop on West syndrome (Commission on Pediatric Epilepsy ILAE, 1992) and recently also by the West Delphi group Consensus (Lux and Osborne, 2004), cases with modified hypsarrhythmia do not need to be reported in dichotomized groups but, where appropriate, a description should be given of the individual modifying features.

Considering the ictal phenomena occurring in West syndrome, we know that it can be characterized by a massive motor phenomena (spasms) and/or by more subtle motor or behavioural manifestations, variably associated to spasms or recurring independently with a variable frequency. As reported in the introduction by Avanzini et al. the typical ictal EEG pattern associated to each spasm is given by a complex and variable wave form including slow and/or sharp transients, variably associated to attenuation and/or brief discharges of fast activity, lasting from one to a few seconds. This fast discharge has been well analyzed by several Authors (Fusco and Vigevano, 1993; Panzica et al., 1999; Kobayashi et al., 2004; Asano et al., 2005) who documented its cortical origin and its relationship with subtle manifestations preceding or accompanying spasms.

The ictal EEG event can be only a part of the above-mentioned patterns and the whole seizure pattern can be the fast activity, alone or superimposed to background attenuation. The subtle seizures are typically associated to attenuation and/or fast activity. The fast activity discharges can be variable in duration (less than 1 sec. or lasting a few sec.), in topography (strictly focal, unilateral or more diffuse), in amplitude (very small or going from 20 to 50-60 µV) and in fast activity frequency (from a brief sinusoidal 12-18 Hz discharge to a more prolonged recruiting discharge). The attenuation can appear as a brief suppression burst or a background attenuation with small fast activity superimposed, recurring with a persisting focal unilateral or diffuse topography or with a more fluctuating topographic expression. Both the fast activity discharges and attenuation can occur independently from spasms and often even in the absence of spasms and can appear related to very subtle, often difficult to detect, motor, autonomic and/or behavioural manifestations *(Figures 6-7)*. In some cases, when recurring subcontinuously, they can realize an unusual long-lasting epileptic status, characterized by a dramatic cognitive and behavioural impairment (Dalla Bernardina et al., 1994). During these statuses obvious paroxysmal abnormalities can be rare or absent and the spasms can remain unrecognized because occurring often randomly and included in the stereotyped gestural automatic motor activities that accompany the severe psychic behavioural disorder.

Therefore it is not surprising that the "interictal" picture, alias the hypsarrhythmia, can be more or less heavily modified or absolutely inhibited not only by the eventual appearance of spasms in clusters, but even by the presence of the above mentioned subtle seizures *(Figures 6, 7)*.

Table I reports the results from the analysis of the electroclinical features at onset in 80 personal cases with infantile spasms:
– in the group showing a typical hypsarrhythmia the subjects presenting spasms without other seizures are predominant (62.5%) with the largest subgroup being the cryptogenic cases (80%);
– in the group showing a modified hypsarrhythmia the subjects only having spasms are very few (7%); likewise, in the group presenting other seizure types the cryptogenic cases (19%) are also very few;
– in the group without hypsarrhythmia the subjects only having spasms are rare (7%) and the cryptogenic cases are rare as well (12%).

It appears that the fluctuation of the hypsarrhythmic pattern and therefore its trend to be modified, is proportional to the presence and frequency of clinically obvious or subtle seizures. While, even if with a low incidence, in the group with modified hypsarrhythmia there are cryptogenic cases (22.5%) and in the group with typical hypsarrhythmia there are symptomatic cases (20%).

An open and intriguing problem remains understanding of the true role of cortical and subcortical structures in the generation of hypsarrhythmia. The interpretation of the hypsarrhythmic pattern, as the result of an "extension" of the paroxysmal activity produced within triggering area favoured by an age-dependent hyperexcitability of wide areas of the cortex, seems supported by the good results obtained by surgical resection of cortical lesions (Shields et al., 1992). We can also give the same meaning to the occurrence during school age of a typical CSWS electroclinical picture in children who had a previous typical West syndrome in the first year of life followed by a good outcome (personal observations).

On the other hand the possible transitory inhibition of the hypsarrhythmic pattern by a partial seizure has been observed in cases of West syndrome and of CSWS (Dalla Bernardina et al., 1978). This inhibition of the paroxysmal activity has induced to hypothesize that the suppression of the interictal activity between spasms during a cluster is sustained by the persisting long lasting focal seizure that triggered the cluster (Gobbi et al., 1987; Dulac, 2001; Pachatz et al., 2003). Yet this explanation of the dramatic suppression of the interictal paroxysmal activity between the spasms during the cluster is probably not satisfactory. The possible occurrence of a pattern characterized by a partial seizure followed by spasms in clusters has been reported by several Authors (Beaussart, 1960; Dalla Bernardina et al., 1984; Gobbi et al., 1987; Yamamoto et al., 1988; Donat and Wright, 1991; Carrazana et al., 1993; Plouin et al., 1993; Viani et al., 1994; Otsuka et al., 1996; Kubota et al., 1999; Pachatz et al., 2003;

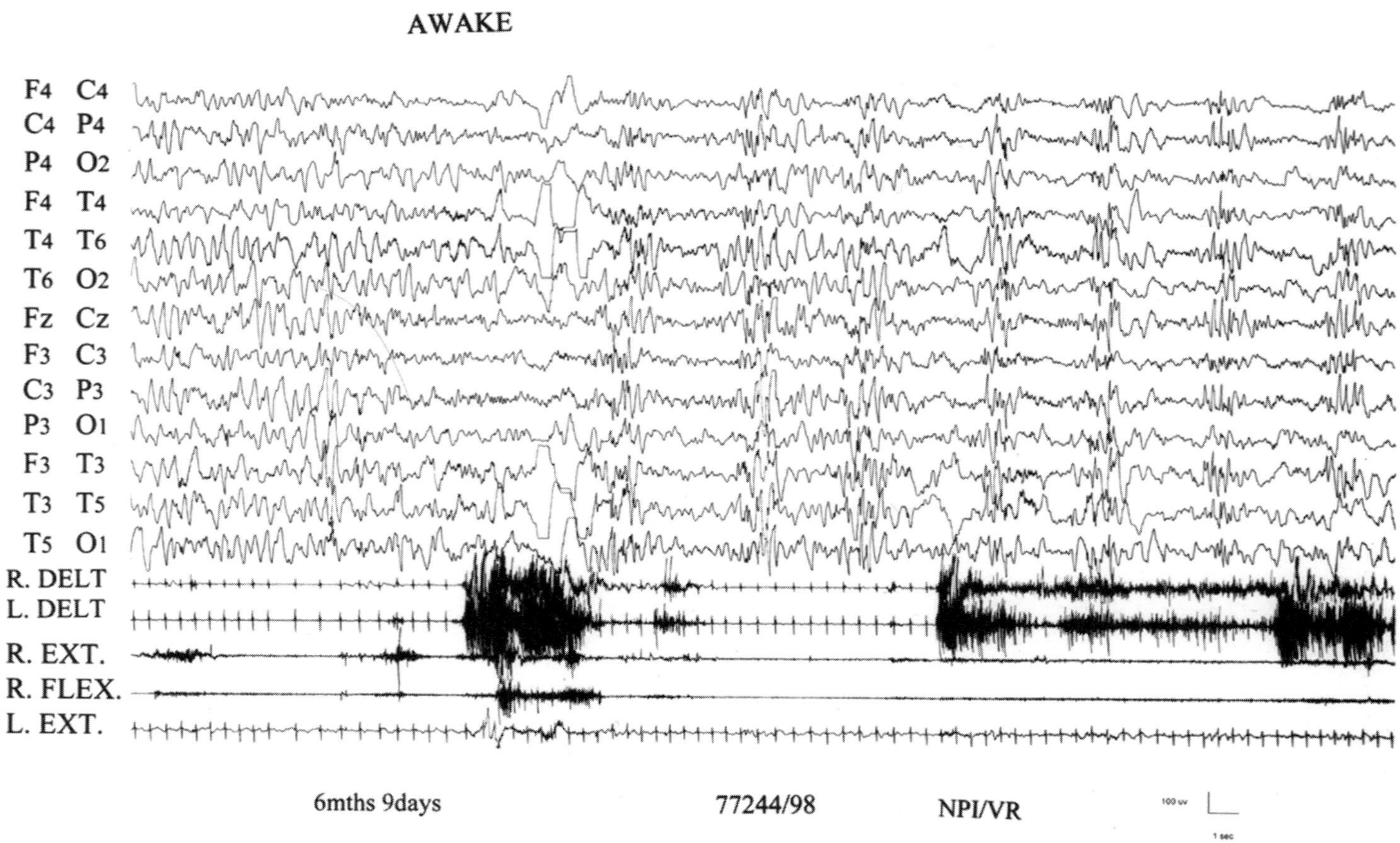

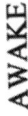

Figure 6. Six months 6 days old girl with normal development suffering from 15 days of infantile spasms in clusters sometimes triggered by a partial seizure involving the left temporo-occipital region, with eyes deviation to the right. Brain MRI is normal. Notice how the brief depression of the EEG activity, often with superimposed small fast activity, sometimes accompanied by a tonic spasm, induces a significant fragmentation of the hypsarrhythmic pattern. Following ACTH treatment the seizures stop. From the age of 5 years rare partial complex seizures reappear and at present (8 years old) they persist rare in spite of VPA treatment. A second MRI performed at the age of 7 did not reveal any abnormality. She has severe learning problems with a borderline IQ.

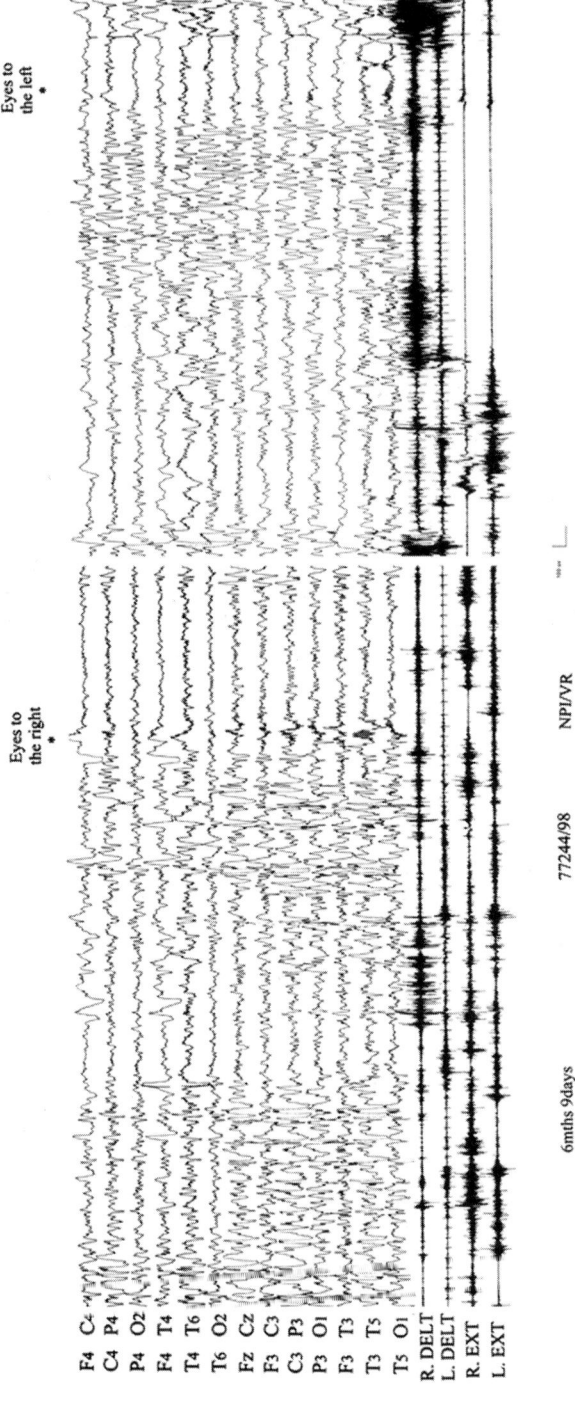

Figure 7. Same case as Figure 6.
The subcontinuous recurrence of subtle seizures inhibits, nearly continuously for long periods, the hypsarrhythmic pattern even outside the clusters of infantile spasms.
Notice the recurrent brief discharges of small fast activity variable in frequency, involving the left temporo-occipital regions. These brief discharges are followed by bursts of diffuse paroxysms of variable duration, in some case abruptly stopped by a brief fast discharge associated with concomitant brief eyes deviation.

Table I. Electroclinical features at onset of 80 personal cases with infantile spasms

Typical hypsarrhythmia 8/80 (10%)				Modified hypsarrhythmia 44/80 (55%)				No hypsarrhythmia 28/80 (35%)			
Only spasms 5/8 (62,5%)		Obvious and subtle partial seizures 3/8 (37,5%)		Only spasms 3/44 (7%)		Obvious and subtle partial seizures 41/44 (93%)		Only spasms 2/28 (7%)		Obvious and subtle partial seizures 26/28 (93%)	
C	S	C	S	C	S	C	S	C	S	C	S
4/5 (80%)	1/5 (20%)	2/3 (66,7%)	1/3 (33,3%)	2/3 (67%)	1/3 (33%)	8/41 (19%)	33/41 (71%)	–	2/2 (100%)	3/26 (12%)	23/26 (88%)

Legend: C = cryptogenic, S = symptomatic

RamachandraNair et al., 2005) and probably, as suggested by Pachatz et al. (2003), it represents a distinct neurophysiologic entity rather than an occasional concomitant occurrence of two independent ictal phenomena. Nevertheless the global inhibition of the hypsarrhythmia during the spasms is similar to that observed in clusters not triggered by a similar partial seizure.

With partial onset seizures the "interictal" paroxysmal abnormalities are partially inhibited for their duration. Only when spasms appear in clusters and there is a concomitant magnification of the diffuse high-voltage slow waves (HVSs) (Kobayashi et al., 2005), the paroxysmal activity results totally suppressed.

This occurs in all cases in which the spasms in clusters are preceded by an increasing trend and followed by a decreasing trend of series of subtle motor or behavioural "ictal" events. The subtle seizures of the increasing phase, progressively modify the "interictal" pattern *(Figures 8, 9)* that progressively reappears during the decreasing phase. But only during the recurrence of massive spasms the interictal paroxysms are completely suppressed *(Figure 10)*. This massive suppression seems therefore induced by a massive inhibition induced by the HVSs or following them. According to these considerations it may result very difficult to distinguish the limits between ictal and interictal status considering all kinds of seizures (spasms, partial seizures, subtle seizures, etc.).

An additional open question is: what is the clinical relevance of hypsarrhythmia *per se*?

The most common definition of West syndrome implies a dichotomous vision for which hypsarrhythmia is an interictal component; the West Delphi group Consensus quotes: "Hypsarrhythmia is an interictal pattern that usually changes during clinical attacks..." Nevertheless West syndrome has been included in the group of epileptic encephalopathies (Engel, 2001), conditions in which the EEG paroxysmal abnormalities themselves are believed to contribute to the progressive disturbance in cerebral functions (Guerrini, 2006).

Several elements show how the hypsarrhythmia can by itself induce cognitive and/or behavioural disorders.

The brief behavioural phenomenon called "psychic awakening" (Launay et al., 1959; Jeavons and Bower, 1974) concomitant with hypsarrhythmia's transitory interruption induced by the spasm is the first evidence of this.

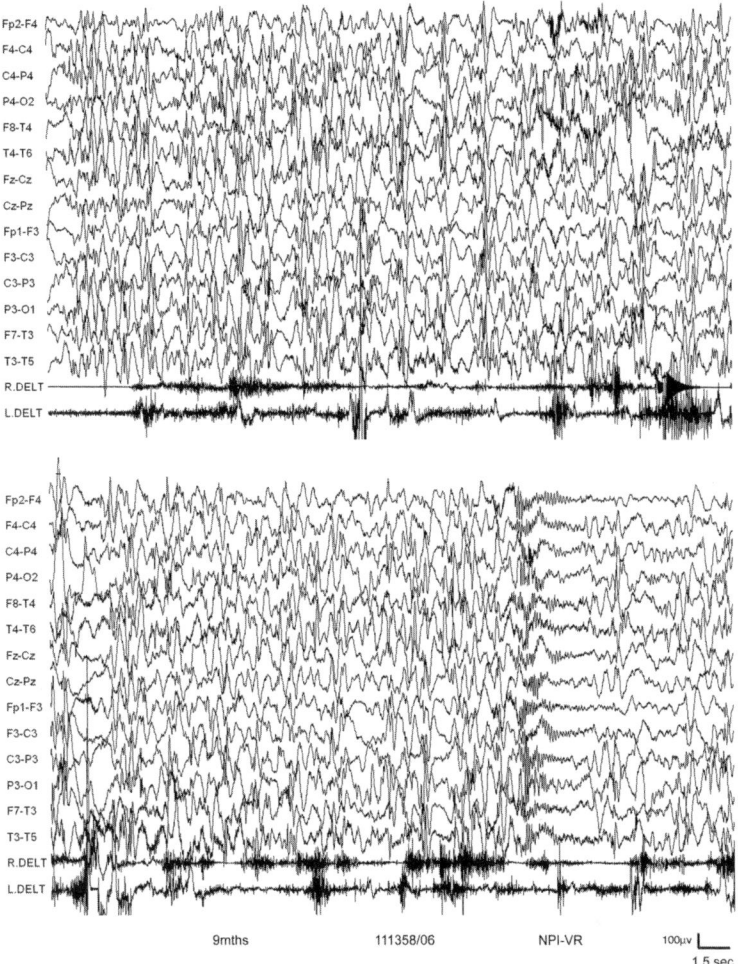

Figure 8. Nine months old girl with mild development delay, without neurological deficits and with normal brain MRI, presenting at the age of 8 months infantile spasms in clusters. Notice how the hypsarrhythmic pattern results only briefly interrupted by isolated spasms.

In addition, several observations have documented how psychomotor deterioration and behavioural disturbances are milder in cases without hypsarrhythmia, either symptomatic or cryptogenic (Jambaqué et al., 1991, 2000; Guzzetta et al., 2002). Higher hypsarrhythmia scores (hypsarrhythmia severity) correlate with higher outcome scores (worse prognosis) (Kramer et al., 1997). Several authors (Matsumoto et al., 1981; Guzzetta et al., 2002; Randò et al., 2005; Baranello et al., 2006) have documented that the neurosensory and cognitive impairment is generally short lasting in cases with transient electroclinical abnormalities.

Finally a prolonged duration of hypsarrhythmia appears to be a negative prognostic factor (Lombroso, 1983; Jayakar and Seshia, 1991; Gaily et al., 1995; Dulac, 2001; Saltik et al., 2002; Kivity et al., 2004; Rho, 2004); very recently Rener-Primec et al.

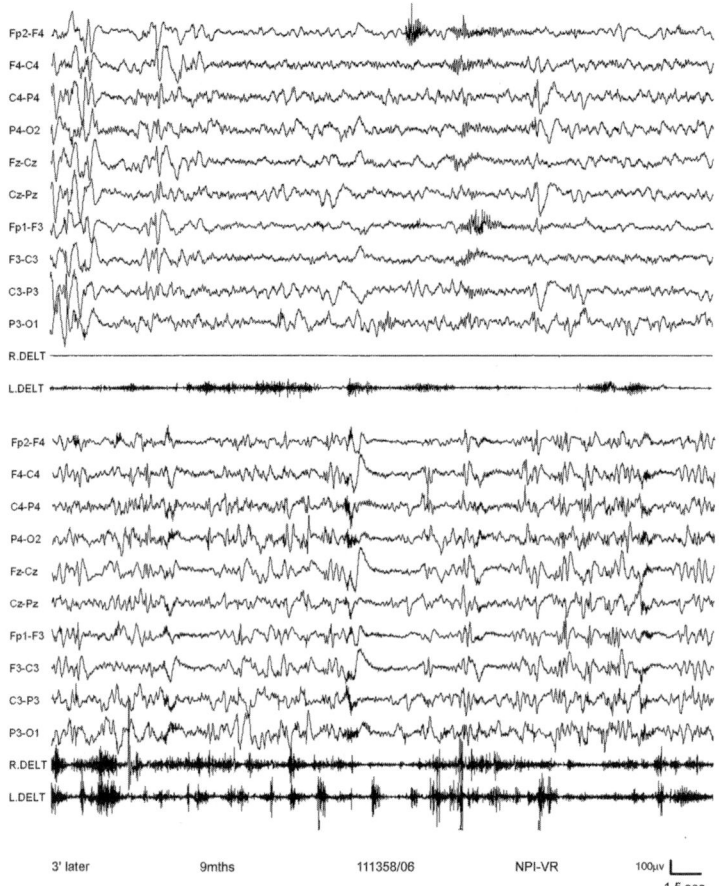

Figure 9. Same EEG recording as Figure 8.
The hypsarrhythmia is inhibited by the appearance of subtle clinically unrecognizable seizures (recurring brief discharges of sinusoidal fast activity involving mainly the left parieto-occipital region); therefore later on with the appearance of brief seizures clinically recognizable by staring and blinking without spasms and related to brief EEG diffuse suppression (below), "interictal" paroxysms constantly reappear after any "ictal" event.

(2006) using a logistic regression model 48 infants with infantile spasms found that after three weeks of hypsarrhythmia the risk of mental retardation increases in both cryptogenic and symptomatic cases. These considerations justify the choice of the West Delphi group Consensus (2004) that considers the resolution of hypsarrhythmia the essential marker of primary electroclinical response together with spasms cessation.

This choice should induce to reconsider hypsarrhythmia as an interictal pattern. As outlined by Dulac (2001) and conceptualized in the International Classification Proposal (Engel, 2001), West syndrome is an intermediary condition between epilepsy with repeated seizures separated by interictal periods and status epilepticus in which the epileptic activity is continuous for a given period of time. In West syndrome

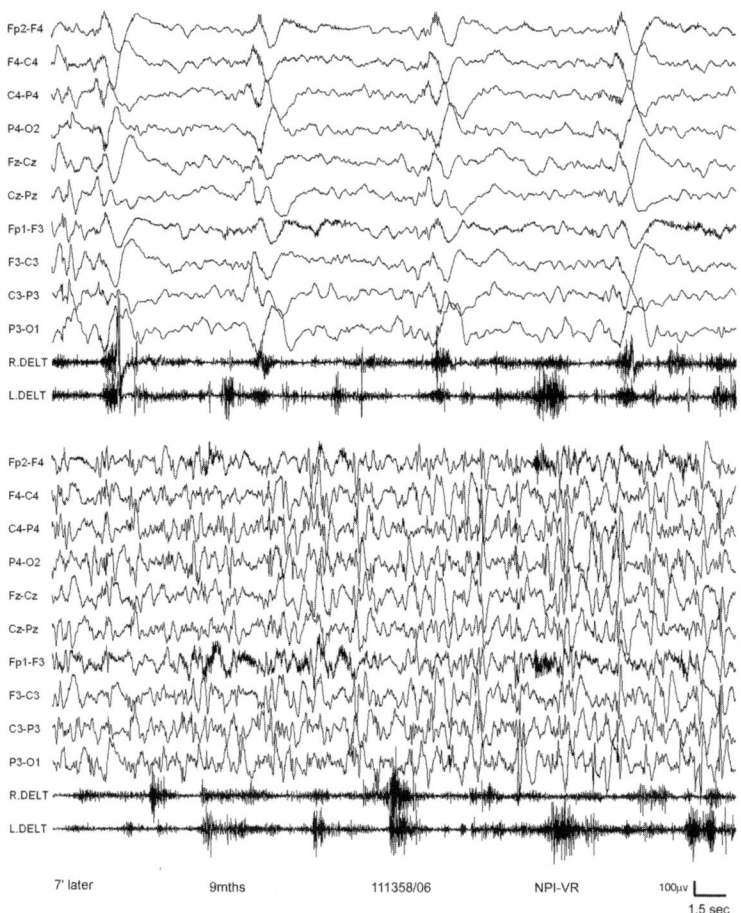

Figure 10. Same EEG recording as Figures 8-9.
Three minutes later with the appearance of spasms (top) and related diffuse slow waves on the EEG, all interictal paroxysms disappear and the background activity remains significantly slowed; 5 minutes later (below) with resolution of spasms the hypsarrhythmic pattern reappears progressively.

seizures can be identified but there is no "interictal" period since the EEG is permanently abnormal with an impact on brain function that reverts in part when the paroxysmal activity comes under control.

In our opinion in West syndrome there are no limits between "interictal" and "ictal"; the entire electroclinical picture represents a continuous ictal status modified by the recurrence of more or less easily detectable "ictal events". The primary therapeutic goal should therefore be the cessation of the electroclinically detectable seizures and the resolution of typical or modified hypsarrhythmia. The more the hypsarrhythmia appears modified or less represented, the stronger the effort must be to recognize subtle seizures and obtain their control. The more the hypsarrhythmia is typical and persistent the more rapidly its resolution should be obtained.

References

Asano E, Juhasz C, Shah A, Muzik O, Chugani DC, Shah J, Sood S, Chugani HT. Origin and propagation of epileptic spasms delineated on electrocorticography. *Epilepsia* 2005; 46 (7): 1086-97.

Baranello G, Rando T, Bancale A, D'Acunto MG, Epifanio R, Frisone MF, Guzzetta A, La Torre G, Mannocci A, Ricci D, Signorini S, Tinelli F, Biagioni E, Veggiotti P, Fazzi E, Mercuri E, Cioni G, Guzzetta F. Auditory attention at the onset of West syndrome: correlation with EEG patterns and visual function. *Brain Dev* 2006; 28 (5): 293-9.

Beaussart M. Encéphalopathie myoclonique du nourrison avec hypsarythmia. Étude EEG avant et aprés traitement par ACTH. *Rev Neurol* 1960; 103: 243-50.

Caraballo RH, Fejerman N, Dalla Bernardina B, Ruggeri V, Cersosimo R, Medina C, Pocieche J. Epileptic spasms in clusters without hypsarrhytmia in infancy. *Epileptic Disord* 2003; 5 (2): 109-13.

Carrazana JE, Lombroso CT, Mikati M, Helmers S, Holmes GL. Facilitation of infantile spasms by partial seizures. *Epilepsia* 1993; 34 (1): 97-109.

Chiron C, Raynaud C, Maziere B, Zilbovicius M, Laflamme L, Masure MC, et al. Changes in regional cerebral blood flow during brain maturation in children and adolescents. *J Nucl Med* 1992; 33: 696-703.

Commission on Pediatric Epilepsy of the International League Against Epilepsy. Workshop on infantile spasms. *Epilepsia* 1992; 33: 195.

Dalla Bernardina B., Tassinari C.A., Dravet C., Bureau M., Beghini G., Roger J. Epilepsie partielle bénigne et état de mal électroencéphalographique pendant le sommeil. *Rev. EEG Neurophysiol.* 1978; 8: 350-3.

Dalla Bernardina B, Colamaria V, Capovilla G, Chiamenti C, Trevisan E, Andrighetto G, et al. Epileptic syndromes and cerebral malformations in infancy: multicentric study. *Boll Lega It Epil* 1984; 45: 46-65.

Dalla Bernardina B, Watanabe K. Interictal EEG: Variations and Pitfalls. In: Dulac O, Chugani HT, Dalla Bernardina B (Eds) *Infantile spasms and West syndrome*. W.B. Saunders Company Ltd., London, 1994: 63-81.

Dalla Bernardina B, Fontana E, Zullini E, Avesani E, Zoccante L, Perez Jimenez A, Giardina L. Unusual partial complex status with autistic behavior in infancy. In: *Abstracts from the European Congress of Epileptology*, Oporto, Portugal september. *Epilepsia* 1994: 6-10.

Dalla Bernardina B, Pérez-Jimènez A, Fontana E, Colamaria V, Piardi F, Avesani E, Santorum E, Grimau-Merino R, Tassinari CA. Electroencephalographic findings associated with cortical dysplasias. In: Guerrini R, Andermann F, Canapicchi R, Roger J, Zifkin BG, Pfanner P. *Dysplasias of cerebral cortex and epilepsy*. Lippincott-Raven, 1996: 235-46.

Donat AF, Wright FS. Simultaneous infantile spasms and partial seizures. *J Child Neurol* 1991; 6 (3): 246-50.

Druckman R, Chao D. Massive spasms in infancy and childhood. *Epilepsia* 1955; 4: 61-72.

Dulac O, Plouin P, Jambaqué I. Predicting favourable outcome in idiopathic West syndrome. *Epilepsia* 1993; 34 (4): 747-56.

Dulac O, Chugani T, Dalla Bernardina B. Overview. In: Dulac O, Chugani HT, Dalla Bernardina B (Eds), Infantile spasms and West Syndrome. London, WB Saunders, 1994: 1-5.

Dulac O. What is West syndrome? *Brain Dev* 2001; 23: 447-52.

Dulac O and Tuxhorn I. Infantile spasms and West syndrome. In: Roger J, Bureau M, Dravet Ch, Genton P, Tassinari CA, Wolf P, *Epileptic syndromes in infancy, childhood and adolescence* (4th ed). Paris: John Libbey, 2005: 53-72.

Engel J. A proposed diagnostic scheme for people with epileptic seizures and with epilepsy: Report of the ILAE Task Force on Classification and Terminology. *Epilepsia* 2001; 42 (6): 796-803.

Fusco L, Vigevano F. Ictal clinical electroencephalographic findings of spasms in West syndrome. *Epilepsia* 1993, 34: 671-8.

Gaily KE, Shewmon DA, Chugani HT, Curran GJ. Asymmetric and asynchronous infantile spasms. *Epilepsia* 1995, 36 (9): 873-82.

Gastaut H, Soulayrol R, Roger J, Pinsard N. *L'encephalopathie myoclonique infantile avec hypsarythmia (syndrome de West)*, Paris: Masson 1964.

Gastaut H. Clinical and electroencephalographical classification of epileptic seizure. *Epilepsia* 1970; 11: 102-13.

Gibbs FA, Gibbs EL. Infantile Spasms. In: *Atlas of electroencephalography*. Cambridge, MA: Addison-Wesley, 1952; 52: 24-30.

Gobbi G, Bruno L, Pini A, Rossi PG, Tassinari CA. Periodic spasms: an unclassified type of epileptic seizure in childhood. *Dev Med Child Neurol* 1987; 29: 766-75.

Guerrini R. Epilepsy in children. *Lancet* 2006; 367: 499-524.

Guzzetta F, Frisone MF, Ricci D, Randò T, Guzzetta A. Development of visual attention in West syndrome. *Epilepsia* 2002; 43 (7): 757-63.

Hrachovy R, Frost J, Jr and P. Kellaway. Sleep characteristics in infantile spasms. *Neurology* 1981; 31: 688-94.

Hrachovy R, Frost J, Jr and P. Kellaway: Hypsarrhythmia. Variations on the Theme. *Epilepsia* 1984; 25 (3); 317-25.

Hrachovy R, and Frost J, Jr. Infantile Epileptic Encephalopathy with Hypsarrhythmia (Infantile Spasms/West Syndrome). *Journal Clin Neurophysiol* 2003; 20 (6): 408-25.

Jambaqué I, Cusmai R, Curatolo P et al. Neuropsychological aspects of tuberous sclerosis: relation to epilepsy and MRI findings. *Dev Med Child Neurol* 1991; 33: 698-705.

Jambaqué I, Chiron C, Dumas C, Mumford J, Dulac O. Mental and behavioural outcome of infantile epilepsy treated by vigabatrin in tuberous sclerosis patients. *Epilepsy Res* 2000; 38: 151-60.

Jayakar PB, Seshia SS. Electrical status epilepticus during slow-wave sleep: a review. *J Clin Neurophysiol* 1991; 8: 299-311.

Jeavons PM, Bower BD. Infantile spasms. In: Vinken PJ, Bruyn GW (eds). *Handbook of clinical neurology*, Vol. 15. The epilepsies. Amsterdam: Elsevier North Holland, 1974: 219-34.

Kellaway P, Frost JD, Hrachovy RA: Infantile spasms. In: Morselli PL et al. (eds), *Antiepileptic drug therapy in pediatrics*. New York: Raven Press. 1983, 115-36.

Kivity S, Lerman P, Ariel R, Danziger Y, Mimouni M, Shinnar S. Long-term cognitive outcomes of a cohort of children with cryptogenic infantile spasms treated with high-dose adrenocorticotropic hormone. *Epilepsia* 2004; 45: 255-62.

Kobayashi K, Oka M, Akiyama T, Inoue T, Abiru K, Ogino T, Yoshinaga H, Ohtsuka Y, Oka E. Very fast rhythmic activity on scalp EEG associated with epileptic spasms. *Epilepsia* 2004; 45 (5): 488-96.

Kobayashi K, Oka M, Inoue T, Ogino T, Yoshinaga H, Ohtsuka Y. Characteristics of slow waves on EEG associated with epileptic spasms. *Epilepsia* 2005; 46: 1098-105.

Kramer U, Sue W, Mikati M.A. Hypsarrhythmia: Frequency of Variant Patterns and Correlation with Etiology and Outcome. *Neurology* 1997; 48 (1): 197-203.

Kubota T, Aso K, Negoro T. Epileptic spasms preceded by partial seizures with a close temporal association. *Epilepsia* 1999; 40: 1572-9.

Launay C, Blanc C, Rebufat-Deschamps M. Spasmes en flexion et hypsarythmia. Mise au point a propos de six observations personnelles. *Presse Med* 1959; 67: 887-90.

Lombroso CT. A prospective study of infantile spasms: clinical and therapeutic correlations. *Epilepsia* 1983; 24: 135-58.

Lux AL, Osborne JP. A proposal for case definitions and outcome measures in studies of infantile spasms and West sindrome: consensus statement of the West Delphi Group. *Epilepsia* 2004; 45 (11): 1416-28.

Matsumoto A, Watanabe K, Negoro T, Iwase K, Hara K, Miyasaki S. Infantile spasms: etiological factors, clinical aspects, and long-term prognosis in 200 cases. *Eur J Pediatr* 1981; 135: 239-44.

Ohtahara S, Yamatogi Y. Severe encephalographic epilepsy in infants: West syndrome. In: Pellock J, Dodson W, Bourgeois B (Eds) *Pediatric Epilepsy: Diagnosis and therapy*, 2nd ed., New York Demos Medical Publishing 2001: 177-92.

Ohtsuka Y, Murashima I, Asano T, Oka E, Ohtahara S. Partial seizures in West syndrome. *Epilepsia* 1996, 37 (11): 1060-7.

Oka M, Kobayashi K, Akyama T, Ogino T, Oka E. A study of spike density on EEG in West syndrome. *Brain Dev* 2004; 26: 105-11.

Pachatz C, Fusco L, Vigevano F. Epileptic spasms and partial seizures as a single ictal event. *Epilepsia* 2003, 44 (5): 693-700.

Pachioli R, Cavazzuti GB: *Le encefalopatie infantili con spasmi ed ipsaritmia*. Minerva Med, 1962.

Panzica F, Franceschetti S, Binelli S, Canafoglia L, Granata T, Avanzini G. Spectral properties of EEG fast activity ictal discharges associated with infantile spasms. *Clinical Neurophysiology* 1999; 110 (4): 593-603.

Plouin P, Dulac O, Jalin C, Chiron C. Twenty-Four-Hour Ambulatory EEG Monitoring in Infantile Spasms. *Epilepsia* 1993; 34 (4): 686-91.

RamachandranNair R, Ochi A, Akiyama T, Buckley DJ, Soman TB, Weiss SK, Otsubo H. Partial Seizures triggering infantile spasms in the presence of a basal ganglia glioma. *Epileptic Disord* 2005; 7 (4): 378-82.

Randò T, Baranello G, Ricci D, Guzzetta A, Tinelli F, Biagioni E, et al. Cognitive competence at the onset of West syndrome: correlation with EEG patterns and visual function. *Dev Med Child Neurol* 2005; 47: 760-5.

Rener-Primec Z, Stare J, Neubauer D. The risk of lower mental outcome in infantile spasms increases after three weeks of hypsarrhythmia duration. *Epilepsia* 2006; 47 (12): 2202-5.

Rho JM. Basic science behind the catastrophic epilepsies. *Epilepsia* 2004; 4 (suppl 5): 5-11.

Saltik S, Kocer N, Dervent A. Informative value of magnetic resonance imaging and EEG in the prognosis of infantile spasms. *Epilepsia* 2002; 43 (3): 246-52.

Shields WD, Shewmon DA, Chugani HT, Peacock W. Treatment of infantile spasms: medical or surgical? *Epilepsia* 1992; 33 (suppl 4) S26-S31.

Sorel L. Le syndrome de West atypique ou incomplet: a propos de 80 observations. *Boll Lega It Epil* 1978; 22/23: 181-2.

Suzuki M, Okumura A, Watanabe K, Negoro T, Hayakawa F, Kato T, et al. The predictive value of electroencephalogram during early infancy for later development of West syndrome in infants with cystic periventricular leukomalacia. *Epilepsia* 2003; 44 (3): 443-6.

Viani F, Romeo A, Mastrangelo M., Viri M. Infantile spasms combined with partial seizures: electro-clinical study of 11 cases. *Ital J Neurol Sci* 1994; 15: 463-71.

Watanabe K, Iwase K, Hara K. The Evolution of EEG Features in Infantile Spasms: a prospective Study. *Development Child Neurology* 1973; 15: 584-96.

Watanabe K, Negoro T, Aso K, Matsumoto A. Reappraisal of Interictal Electroencephalograms in Infantile Spasms. *Epilepsia* 1993; 34 (4): 679-85.

Yamamoto N, Watanabe K, Negoro T, Furune S, Takahashi I, Nomura K, Matsumoto A: Partial seizures evolving to infantile spasms. *Epilepsia* 1988; 29 (1): 34-40.

Epileptic spasms: ictal patterns

Federico Vigevano[1], Paolo Montaldo[2], Nicola Specchio[1], Lucia Fusco[1]

[1] Division of Neurology, Bambino Gesù Children's Hospital, IRCCS Rome, Italy
[2] Division of Pediatrics, Annunziata Hospital, Naples, Italy

---

Epileptic spasms are a severe type of epileptic seizure both because they are often drug resistant and also because they are frequently associated with an epileptic encephalopathy with serious repercussions on cognitive and psychomotor development.

Epileptic spasms are seizures observed in children with focal, hemispheric or diffuse cerebral lesions. At times no obvious cerebral lesion can be found and psychomotor development is normal until the onset of the spasms. These cases, according to the old classification of epilepsies (Commission on Classification, 1989), are classified as "cryptogenic". This distinction is useful for prognostic purposes: the "symptomatic" cases are in fact resistant to treatment in about two thirds of the cases; in the "cryptogenic" seizures can be controlled in around 85-90% of the cases.

There has been much discussion about the pathogenesis of the epileptic spasms and in particular whether it is a phenomenon with a "cortical" or "subcortical" origin.

The study of the ictal pattern of spasms is helpful when attempting to discover where the spasm originates. This knowledge could be particularly useful in cases where neurosurgical treatment is an option.

■ Clinical characteristics

The epileptic spasm is a particular type of seizures included as such only in the last Classification of Seizures and Epilepsies in 2001 (Engel, 2001). Previously, in the Classification of Seizures of 1985 (Commission on Classification, 1985), epileptic spasms had not been recognized as distinct seizure type. In the Classification of Epileptic Syndromes (Commission on Classification, 1989), the epileptic spasm was mentioned as the main seizure type of an age-dependent generalized cryptogenic or symptomatic epileptic syndrome, the West syndrome, to which epileptic spasms historically belonged.

It is now well admitted that epileptic spasms, a peculiar distinct seizure type, belong to many different syndromic entities, of which West syndrome is only the most well known.

West syndrome is an age-dependent syndrome of the first year of life, characterized by epileptic spasms, hypsarrhythmic EEG and psychomotor regression. When epileptic spasms, with or without psychomotor regression, are associated to EEG changes other than hypsarrhythmia it is preferable to diagnose *Infantile Spasms Syndrome*, as suggested by the consensus on Infantile Spasms and West Syndrome of West Delphi Group (Lux and Osborne, 2004).

Another condition in infancy in which epileptic spasms have been reported is that of *epileptic spasms following focal seizures*. These are focal epilepsies, mainly of symptomatic origin, in which for unknown reasons each focal seizure is followed by a cluster of epileptic spasms.

In order to describe the ictal patterns of epileptic spasms we will consider both the clinical and the neurophysiological aspects. According to the ILAE Task Force on Classification and Terminology (Engel, 2001) the spasm is described from the clinical point of view as: *"A sudden flexion, extension or mixed extension-flexion of predominantly proximal and truncal muscles which is usually more sustained than a myoclonic movement but not as sustained as a tonic seizure i.e. about one sec."*

The definition proposed by the West Delphi Group (Lux and Osborne, 2004) is very similar: *"Clinical spasms: Brief movements of the head, trunk, and limbs or sometimes of the head, trunk, or limbs alone... have a longer duration than the movements of myoclonus, and they are shorter than the movements associated with a tonic seizure. Thus duration is about one second."*

These definitions put the emphasis mainly on the motor manifestations that characterize the spasm. As pointed out by Fusco and Vigevano in 1993, definition of epileptic spasms should take in account the polygraphic elements that distinguish a spasm from a myoclonus or a tonic seizure. As can be seen in *Figure 1*, a myoclonic jerk is a rapid shock-like contraction of limited duration, while the tonic seizure is a prolonged muscle contraction of growing intensity. The true spasm consists of a characteristic muscular contraction that lasts from 1 to 2 sec. and reaches a peak more slowly than a myoclonic jerk but more rapidly than a tonic seizure. The electromyographic aspect is thus different from a myoclonic or a tonic event and resembles a rhombus.

Kellaway et al. (1979) analyzed more than 5,000 ictal spasms in 24 children and grouped them, according to the predominant features, as flexor, extensor, and mixed flexor-extensor types. Flexor spasms consist of flexion of the neck, trunk, arms, and legs. Spasms of the muscles of the upper limbs result either in symmetrical adduction of the arms in a self-hugging motion or in adduction of the arms to either side of the head with the arms flexed at the elbow. Extensor spasms consist of a predominance of extensor muscle contractions producing abrupt extension of the neck and trunk with extensor abduction or adduction of the arms, legs, or both. Mixed flexor-extensor spasms include flexion of the neck, trunk and arms and symmetrical extension of the legs or flexion of the legs and extension of the arms with varying degrees of flexion

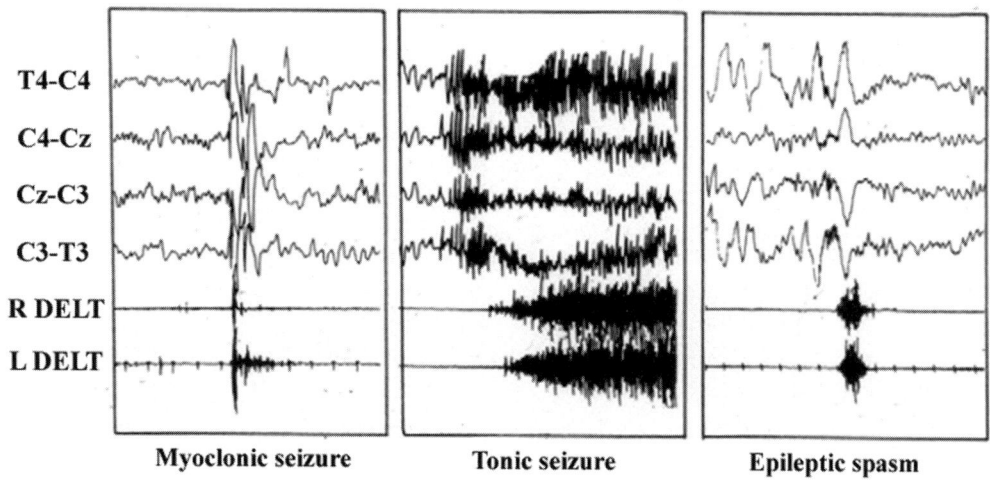

modified from Fusco L and Vigevano F. Epilepsia 1993;34(4):671-8.

Figure 1. Polygraphic recording of myoclonic seizure, tonic seizure and epileptic spasm.
The duration of the epileptic spasm is intermediate between the myoclonic and tonic seizure. The morphology of the EMG trace of the spasm shows a rhomboidal aspect; this correlate with the diffuse slow wave on the EEG traces and appear clearly distinct with the myoclonic and tonic EMG pattern.

of the neck and trunk. The authors described the muscle activity typically consisting of two separated phases: an initial phasic component not exceeding two seconds, and a subsequent tonic contraction lasting from 2-10 seconds.

Fusco and Vigevano (1993), who analysed a more selected population of infantile spasms in West syndrome, with the exclusion of children with lateralized hypsarrhythmia or without hypsarrhythmia, found, among 955 epileptic spasms recorded in 36 infants, that the mean duration of a single spasm, calculated on the basis of EMG recording from the deltoid muscles, was 1,25 seconds in cryptogenic and 1,56 seconds in the symptomatic group, and however none recorded spasm lasted longer than 2,40 seconds.

Reviewing the data collected by Kellaway, at the light of these last results, we can conclude that only the phasic component of the spasm described by Kellaway corresponds to the epileptic spasm as studied by Fusco and Vigevano. This could explain also the differences the two groups found in the EEG counterpart of the epileptic spasms, as the inclusion criteria of studied events was very different. Successively, Fusco and Vigevano (1994) also described more prolonged epileptic spasms as a different seizure type, and they proposed to keep apart these events from true epileptic spasms and suggested to call them tonic-spasm seizures.

Whether the spasm is flexor, extensor or mixed has little diagnostic value as it depends on the child's posture at the moment of the ictal event. In fact different patterns could be found in the same child even within the same cluster. This aspect of the phenomenon has probably been overemphasized in the past. What is important is whether the spasm is symmetrical or asymmetrical, bilateral or unilateral, with or without focal signs *(Figure 2)*. As pointed out by Fusco and Vigevano in 1993, and as other authors have already reported (Kellaway *et al.*, 1979) all these elements indicate a symptomatic origin. Further more prolonged epileptic spasms, *i.e.* more than one second but less than two appear to belong to symptomatic etiology, suggesting that this simple clinical criteria could be, useful to make a first differentiation between cryptogenic and symptomatic etiology. However, although asymmetric spasms, or focal signs recognizable during a spasm, strongly indicate the existence of a cerebral lesion, symmetric spasms could be present both in cryptogenic and symptomatic patients.

Based on these observations, the symmetry or asymmetry and the synchrony or asynchrony of the motor component, and the presence of subtle focal signs, are the more significant elements to suggest a symptomatic etiology. To obtain these prognostic indicators it is fundamental to perform a video-EEG study during a cluster of spasms. Video-EEG should be carried out with polygraphic recording of at least the deltoid muscles, respiration and ECG. Some focal signs as eye deviation toward one side or minimal asynchronies could be missed without a video-EEG study. The recognition of these clinical signs implies different etiological factors and sometimes the suspicion of a cerebral focal lesion that could be missed in the first steps of the diagnostic procedure.

A common feature of infantile spasms is that they typically occur in clusters and the intensity and frequency of the spasms in each cluster may increase in a crescendo fashion, peaking and then slowly decreasing in intensity. The number of spasms per

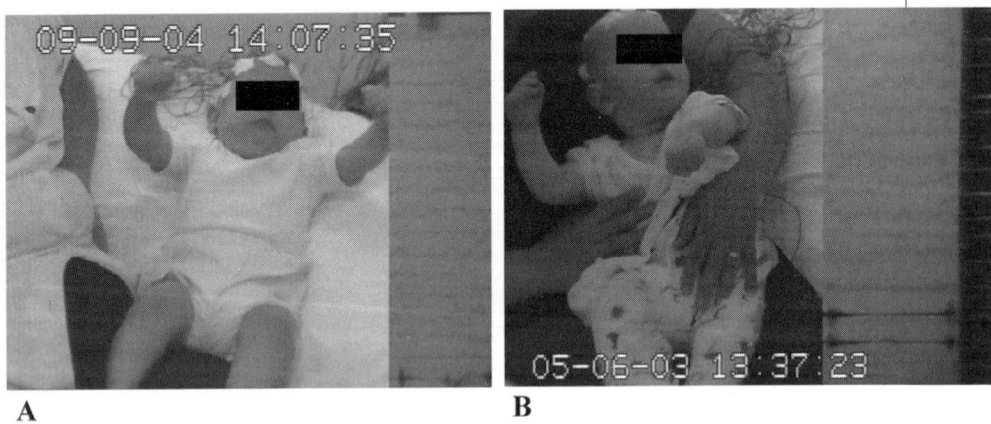

Figure 2. A. Symmetric epileptic spasm in a 7 months old infant with a cryptogenic West Syndrome. **B.** Asymmetric epileptic spasm in a 8 months old infant with West Syndrome symptomatic of right porencephaly as result of perinatal cerebral hemorrhag.

cluster varies considerably with some clusters having as many as 150 spasms. The number of clusters per day also varies. Clusters usually occur shortly after awakening but they can also begin when fully awake or during sleep.

Bisulli *et al.* (2002), whose research has been dedicated to the polygraphic analysis of the "motor" component of the spasm, have come to the conclusion that the sequence of activation of the different muscles is variable and does not follow the rostrocaudal activation pattern. These authors also recognize in spasms two different components, a phasic and a tonic one variably mixed. The four reported patients however all had severe brain malformations and all presented with epileptic encephalopathy and refractory infantile spasms. Whatever the case, the phasic and tonic components of each epileptic spasm were considered two different events, developing in a variable order, one or the other missing. Even though different spasms seem clinically very similar, the first activated muscle could vary in different spasms also in the same patient. Even the latencies of muscle activation could vary among the different spasms, as well as the sequence of muscle activation. Thus the "spasm" does not have the characteristics of a phenomenon of "cortical" origin, such as for example the "cortical myoclonus".

As a matter of fact a careful clinical observation of epileptic spasms has shown that the spasm is at times preceded or associated with *focal clinical signs* such as staring, ocular movements, facial grimaces or *autonomic manifestations* such as tachycardia, pallor or cyanosis. Some of these manifestations, in particular staring, ocular deviations and facial grimaces probably have a cortical origin in contrast to the motor component of the spasm. Moreover, such subtle focal sings can be observed as isolated signs of spasms or at the beginning of a cluster of spasms. In fact if we observe a cluster of spasms we see that there are some ictal events in which the movement of the limbs and trunk is very slight or almost absent and the critical signs are limited to yawning, gasping, facial grimacing and staring. These minimal clinical events are called *"subtle spasms"* (Lux and Osborne, 2004).

■ EEG characteristics

Reviewing 5,042 epileptic spasms in 24 infants, Kellaway *et al.* (1979) identified 11 different ictal patterns. A generalized slow wave pattern, followed or not by a period of voltage attenuation was present in 48,8% of the seizures. A generalized sharp and slow-wave complex followed or not by a period of voltage attenuation was seen in 30,6%. These two patterns were the most represented. Although each particular type of EEG pattern did not correlate closely with a specific type of clinical events, they themselves admitted that motor spasms were most frequently associated with a high-voltage generalized slow transient, while "arrest" attacks were typically accompanied by periods of voltage attenuation with superimposed fast activity.

In 1993 Fusco and Vigevano confirmed that different types of ictal EEG patterns exist; such as a wide positive-vertex slow wave, a fast activity of brief duration and more rarely a desynchronization of electrical activity. Nevertheless, when they looked at the EEG counterpart of motor spasms, invariably they identified a wide positive-vertex slow wave. While the slow wave was present in all cases and always coincided with the motor manifestation of the spasm, the fast activity occurred alone or preceded or followed by the slow wave. When it was alone, or when it preceded the slow wave, the main associated clinical feature was a motionless stare. The fast activity seems therefore to be the EEG equivalent of the "subtle spasms". In a cluster of spasms the fast activity could be the first indicator of an incoming cluster, and at the beginning it can be associated with absence of evident clinical signs, these being completely subclinical. Then minimal signs such opening of the eyes could appear as "subtle spasms", finally motor phenomena are clearly evident and fast activity is followed by the slow wave. The high voltage slow wave seems thus to coincide with the phasic component of the spasm (*Figure 3*).

Lastly, when the fast activity follows the slow wave it was found to coincide with the tonic phase of the motor manifestation. This pattern is very obvious in so-called "tonic spasms" seizures a type of epileptic spasm observed mainly in patients who are drug resistant and have had seizures for a long time. The "tonic spasm" is in fact a seizure in which the classic movement of flexion of the limbs and trunk is followed by a brief tonic phase. In coincidence with the spasm the EEG shows the wide slow wave while a train of fast activity is recorded in coincidence with the tonic phase (*Figure 4*).

Kobayashi et al. (2005) carefully analysed the high voltage slow wave (HVS) associated with the spasm, demonstrating that this can also occur symmetrically in symptomatic cases with focal lesions. Only rarely does the wide slow wave occur asymmetrically and the distribution of HVS coincides with the more pathologically involved hemisphere.

Previously, Kobayashi et al. (2004) had analysed the fast activity recorded with scalp EEG concomitantly with the spasm, stressing the correlation between a possible asymmetry and the localization of the lesion. According to Kobayashi et al. (2004) this fast activity thus reflects the neocortical involvement in the genesis of the spasm: the latter could be the result of a particular interaction between cortical and subcortical structures.

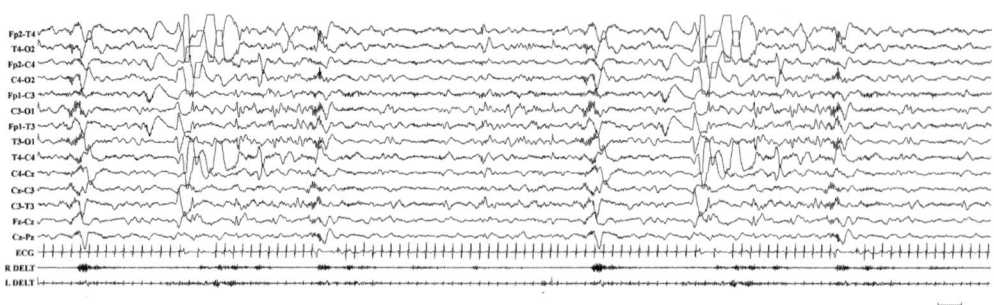

Figure 3. Epileptic spasms in cluster in a 8 months old infant with symptomatic Infantile Spasms Syndrome.
Each ictal event is characterised by diffuse fast activity, more evident over the left central and temporal regions, followed by diffuse high amplitude slow wave. The EMG activity strictly correlate with the slow component.

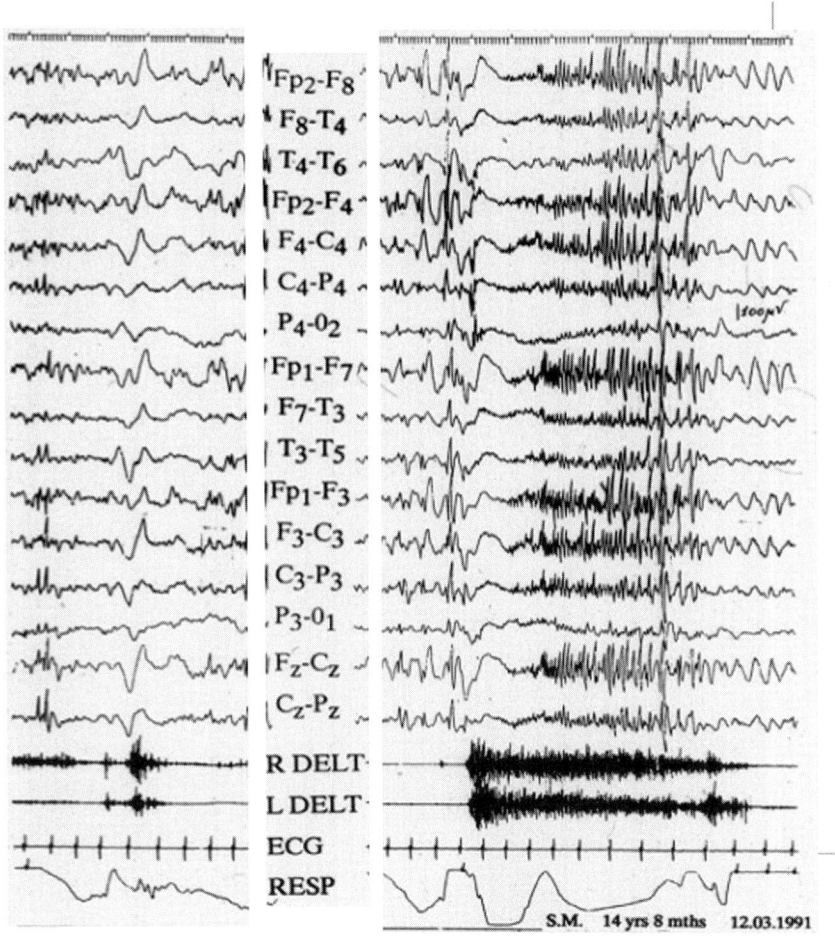

Figure 4. Epileptic spasm (left) and tonic-spasm seizure (right) in a 14 years old boy with a history of drug resistant infantile spasms since the first year of life.
During the same EEG investigation we have recorded a symmetric epileptic spasm (left) with an EEG counterpart characterized by a diffuse slow wave with a maximum peak over the bilateral central regions and a tonic-spasm seizure (right) with an ictal EEG characterized by a diffuse high amplitude slow wave, followed by a fast rhythm of increasing amplitude. The EMG traces of deltoid muscles show the spasm (left) and the tonic-spasm seizure (right), this characterised in the initial part by a rhomboidal aspect as for spasm followed by a persistence of muscular tone which correspond to the tonic phase.

The fast activity seems therefore also to have a localizing value since it has a greater correlation with the localization of the lesion than that of the wide slow wave.

Electrocorticography studies carried out on patients with symptomatic resistant epileptic spasms, candidates for neurosurgical treatment, are also particularly interesting. Asano *et al.* (2005) have demonstrated that in coincidence with the spasm, fast activity sometimes preceded by a spike leading is recorded at cortical level. This data

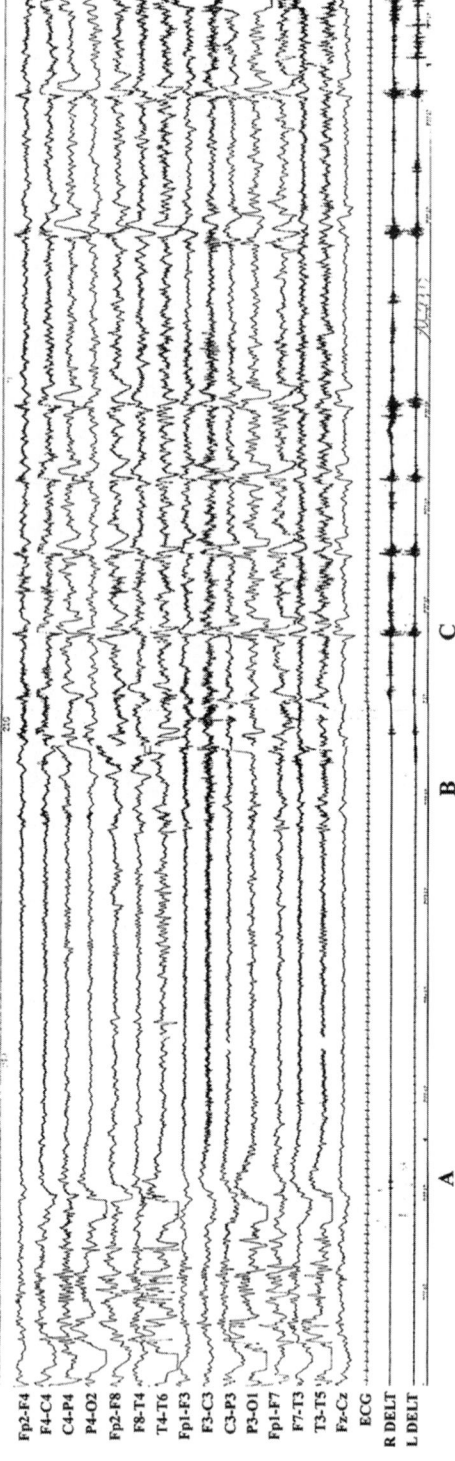

Figure 5. Partial seizure followed by a cluster of spasms in a 5 months old infant. This child was affected by focal epilepsy symptomatic of a right temporal lobe tumour.
Partial seizure started on awakening over the posterior right temporal regions (A) with flattening followed by rhythmic theta activity with the maximum peak over T4, T6 electrodes. Clinically the child opened the eyes and then presented left eye and head deviation associated to left arm hypertonia. Partial seizures ended (B) and promptly symmetrical epileptic spasms appeared (C).

seems to confirm that there is a cortical trigger in epileptic spasms. One more argument in favor of the presence of a cortical trigger derives from the fact that in surgical cases the cortical resection leads to the disappearance of seizures.

Finally, it is worth remembering that spasms can appear in close relation with other types of seizures, particularly with partial seizures. This is a rare event that occurs predominantly during the first year of life. This phenomenon has been reported in infants with a high prevalence of brain structural abnormalities, thus it could be considered distinctive for symptomatic etiology (Ohtsuka et al., 1996). Pachatz et al. (2003) reported epileptic spasms and partial seizures as a single ictal event in 13 patients. The occurrence of epileptic spasms and partial seizures in close temporal association was a transitory phenomenon in all children, as the duration was consistently less than 6 months, representing probably an age-dependent phenomenon. Although the authors described three different pattern of association between epileptic spasms and partial seizures (the cluster could follow, coincide or precede the partial event), we believe that only the pattern of partial seizure constantly followed by a cluster of spasms clarify the role of the cortex in facilitating the epileptic spasms through descending electrical volley to the brainstem *(Figure 5)*. The phenomenon is related to different etiologies and the outcome is not constantly unfavourable, as previously believed (Kubota T et al., 1999). Partial seizures followed by epileptic spasms seem to be a phenomenon probably based on abnormal functional interaction between cortex and subcortical structures and therefore represents a distinct neurophysiological entity rather than the occasional occurrence of two indipendent ictal phenomena.

■ Conclusions

The study of the ictal patterns of epileptic spasms can provide important information regarding etiology and prognosis of the underling epileptic syndrome. Simple clinical observation with attention to the presence of asymmetry or asynchrony in muscle contraction and focal signs can indicate a symptomatic etiology.

Neurophysiological research seems to indicate that the motor phenomenon "spasm" has a subcortical nature. However, there are clinical, EEG and ECoG evidences that indicate a cortical trigger. This theory is supported by the success achieved with cortical resection in patients with drug-resistant spasms.

We can therefore confirm that epileptic spasms seem to derive from a particular age-dependent cortical-subcortical interaction.

References

Asano E, Juhasz C, Shah A et al. Origin and propagation of epileptic spasms delineated on electrocorticography. *Epilepsia* 2005; 46: 1086-97.

Bisulli F, Volpi L, Meletti S et al. Ictal pattern of EEG and muscular activation in symptomatic infantile spasms: a videopolygraphic and computer analysis. *Epilepsia* 2002; 43: 1559-63.

Commission on Classification and Terminology of the International League Against Epilepsy. Proposal for classification of epilepsies and epileptic syndrome. *Epilepsia* 1985; 26: 268-78.

Commission on Classification and Terminology of the International League Against Epilepsy. Proposal of revised classification of epilepsies and epileptic syndromes. *Epilepsia* 1989; 30: 389-99.

Engel J Jr. A proposed diagnostic scheme for people with epileptic seizures and with epilepsy: report of the ILAE Task Force on Classification and Terminology. *Epilepsia* 2001; 42: 796-803.

Fusco L and Vigevano F. Ictal clinical elettroencephalographic findings of spasms in West syndrome. *Epilepsia* 1993; 34: 671-8.

Fusco L and Vigevano F. Tonic spasms: a particular type of unreported seizure. *Epilepsia* 1994; 35 (S7): 87.

Kellaway P, Hrachovy RA, Frost JD, Zion T. Precise characterization and quantification of infantile spasms. *Ann Neurol* 1979; 6: 214-8.

Kobayashi K, Ok M, Akiyama T *et al*. Very fast rhythmic activity on scalp EEG associated with epileptic spasms. *Epilepsia* 2004; 45: 488-96.

Kobayashi K, Ok M, Inoue T, Ogino T, Yoshinaga H, Ohtsuka Y. Characteristics of slow waves on EEG associated with epileptic spasms. *Epilepsia* 2005; 46: 1098-105.

Kubota T, Aso K, Negoro T, *et al*. Epileptic spasms preceded by partial seizures with a close temporal association. *Epilepsia* 1999; 40: 1572-9.

Lux AL and Osborne JP. A proposal for case definition and outcome measures in studies of Infantile Spasms and West Syndrome: consensus statement of the West Delphi Group. *Epilepsia* 2004; 45: 1416-28.

Ohtsuka Y, Murashima I, Asano T, *et al*. Partial seizures in West syndrome. *Epilepsia* 1996; 37: 1060-7.

Pachatz C, Fusco L, Vigevano F. Epileptic spasms and partial seizures as a single ictal event. *Epilepsia* 2003; 44: 693-700.

Spasms outside West syndrome

Giuseppe Gobbi[1], Daniele Frattini[1], Antonella Boni[1], Elvio Della Giustina[2], Gianna Bertani[2]

[1] *Child Neurology Unit, Department of Neuroscience – Maggiore "C.A. Pizzardi" Hospital, Bologna, Italy*
[2] *Child Neurology Unit, Paediatric Department, Arcispedale Santa Maria Nuova, Reggio Emilia, Italy*

In 2004 the Consensus Statement of the West Delphi Group proposed using the term *clinical spasm* to describe a paroxysmal clinical phenomenon not necessarily epileptic in nature and reserving the term *epileptic spasm* to describe an epileptic ictal event. *Clinical spasms* were described as brief (about one second) and synchronous movements of the head, trunk and limbs or sometimes of the head, trunk and limbs alone. Movements may be flexor or extensor or a mixture and they may be symmetrical (Lux AL, 2004). In 2003, Caraballo *et al.* summarised a large list of *Non-Epileptic Clinical Spasms* including abdominal pain (colic), benign neonatal sleep myoclonus, hyperekplexia, Sandifer syndrome, early breath-holding spells and syncopal attacks, adverse reactions or intolerance to exogenous agents, paroxysmal dystonia and choreoathetosis (paroxysmal torticollis, benign infantile dystonia), increased Moro reflex and attacks of opisthotonus, self-gratification or masturbation-like episodes, benign paroxysmal tonic upward gaze, shuddering attacks, Fejerman syndrome (benign myoclonus of early infancy), and tonic reflex seizure of early infancy (Caraballo *et al.*, 2003). Repetitive sleep starts as an unusual non-epileptic manifestation have been described, as well (Fusco *et al.*, 1999).

The *epileptic spasm* (ES) is an epileptic clinical spasm associated with an interictal and ictal EEG consistent with diagnosis of epilepsy, and not necessarily hypsarrhytmia or any specific pattern (Lux AL, 2004). In 1993 Fusco and Vigevano clearly defined the polygraphic semiology of the ES: "... the true spasm consists of a characteristic muscular contraction that lasts from one to 2 seconds, and reaches a peak more slowly than a myoclonic jerk, but more rapidly than a tonic seizure. It then decreases equally quickly and appears polygraphically as a kind of rhombus..." (Fusco and Vigevano, 1993). In 2001, the report of the ILAE Task Force on Classification and Terminology (Blume WT, 2001) defined the ES as a sudden flexion, extension, or mixed extension-flexion of predominantly proximal and truncal muscles which is usually more sustained than a myoclonic movement but not so sustained as a tonic seizure (*i.e.* about one second). Limited forms may occur: grimacing, head nodding. ES frequently occuring in clusters.

In the past, ES were called Infantile Spasms (IS) and were usually considered a type of seizure, specific of the West Syndrome (WS). Several Commissions of the International League Against Epilepsy (ILAE) commissions and workshops have been set up to define and classify the WS, and Proposals from the ILAE Commissions on Classification and Terminology in 1985 and 1989 (Commission on Classification and Terminology of the International League Against Epilepsy, 1985; 1989) suggested that WS is an epileptic disorder characterized by three distinctive features: IS, hypsarrhythmia and arrest or regression of psychomotor development. IS usually appear in clusters and have an age-dependent onset mostly between 4 and 7 months. Differently, in 1991 the workshop of the ILAE Commission on Paediatric Epilepsy suggested that IS "transcends age groups and may occur in infancy or childhood", and suggested to name them ES and to reserve the term IS for spasms which start within the first year of life (Commission on Pediatric Epilepsy of the International League Against Epilepsy, 1992). In fact, reviewing the literature, several articles demonstrated that there were about 2-6% of patients with WS begin after the age of one year (Hrachovy and Frost, 1989), and that ES might have a late onset in patients with localization-related epilepsies (Gobbi et al., 1987) and Lennox Gastaut syndrome (LGS) (Boniver et al., 1987; Donat and Wright, 1991b; Mizukawa et al., 1992). ES might also continue to be present in patients with LGS, which had evolved from a previous WS (Shigematsu et al., 1987). More recently, it has been confirmed the evidence of late-onset ES (Bednarek et al., 1998; Wirrell and Tong 1998), and it has even been hypothesized the existence of an epileptic encephalopathy characterized by cryptogenic late-onset ES (Eisermann et al., 2006). Thus, depending on age at onset, ES are defined as IS when spasms start during the first year of life, and Late-Onset Epileptic Spasms (LOES) when spasms start later.

Infantile Spasms and *late-onset epileptic spasms* may not fit the typical pattern of WS, and may not be specific of WS. This is the case of patients with Aicardi syndrome and agyria-pachygyria brain malformations (Chevrie and Aicardi, 1986; Aicardi J, 1991), with hemimegalencephaly (Vigevano et al., 1996), with Ohtahara Syndrome (Ohtahara et al., 1992), and patients with an early onset lesional localization-related epilepsy due to a clastic lesion, tuberous sclerosis or cortical dysplasia. In these cases the cluster of spasms may be preceded by a focal ictal event (Gobbi et al., 1987 and 1996; Yamamoto et al., 1988; Donat and Wright, 1991a; Carrazana et al., 1993; Ohtsuka et al., 1996; Pachatz et al., 2003). This type of seizure has been called *"Periodic Spasms"* (Gobbi et al., 1987) or "simultaneous seizure" (Donat and Wright, 1991a; Ohtsuka et al., 1996). Otsuka Y (1998) and Otsuka et al. (2001) suggested to divide these spasms outside WS into three groups: 1) early-onset spasms in cluster and atypical EEG features in refractory epilepsies such as Aicardi syndrome, early myoclonic encephalopathy, and Ohtahara syndrome; 2) spasms in cluster at the age of 2-3 years or above, appearing in cases of generalized epilepsies; 3) spasms in cluster appearing in cases of localization-related epilepsies.

Epileptic spasms outside West syndrome

Epileptic Spasms Outside West Syndrome (ESOWS) are the spasms that do not fit the standard pattern of WS (Ohtsuka Y, 2001).

ESOWS may start *before* the age of one year, and may be cryptogenic or lesional. ESOWS may also start *after* the age of one year, and may be found in the case of cryptogenic or lesional partial epilepsies and epileptic encephalopathies.

ESOWS starting before the age of 1 year

Cryptogenic ESOWS

This is a rare condition reported in patients affected by clusters of spasms without hypsarrhytmia or modified hypsarrhytmia, and with normal neuroimaging, normal neurometabolic investigations. Focal seizures may be also associated. Spasms are usually refractory to AEDs, but there is not evolution into LGS (Caraballo *et al.*, 2003).

Lesional ESOWS

Epileptic Spasms are the typical ictal event of the Early-infantile epileptic encephalopathy with suppression bursts or Ohtahara's syndrome (Ohtahara *et al.*, 1992), of Early Myoclonic Encephalopathy (Aicardi J, 1992), of the Aicardi syndrome (Chevrie and Aicardi, 1986; Ohtsuka *et al.*, 1993), of cases with cortical malformations such as diffuse pachygyria, focal cortical dysplasia, polymicrogyria, hemimegalencephaly, and of Tuberous Sclerosis (Aicardi J, 1991; Vigevano *et al.*,1996; Ohtsuka *et al.*, 1996; Ohtsuka *et al.*, 1999; Donat and Wright, 1991a; Pini *et al.*, 1996), as well as of cases with acquired clastic lesions, such as perinatal anoxic-ischemic encephalopathy (Gobbi *et al.* 1987).

In cryptogenic and lesional patients, partial seizures and spasms may co-exist all over the evolution, and partial seizures usually start earlier than the spasms. More frequently in these patients the cluster of spasms is preceded by a focal ictal event (Gobbi *et al.*, 1987; Donat and Wright, 1991a; Carrazana *et al.*, 1993; Otsuka *et al.*, 1996; Pachatz *et al.*, 2003). Interictal EEG usually shows multifocal spikes, sometimes associated with diffuse spike-waves. *Polygraphic recordings* showed that the spasms are often asymmetric and concomitant with an EEG complex characterized by a slow wave with superimposed fast activity. The ictal focal event preceding the cluster of spasms may consist of a focal EEGraphic discharge, or an electroclinical event characterized by a partial motor seizure, or a hemiclonic seizure or a partial complex seizure (Gobbi *et al.*, 1987; Gobbi *et al.*, 1996; Ohtsuka Y., 1998). Otsuka *et al.* (1996) and Donat and Wright (1991a) suggested to call this combination of focal ictal events followed by a cluster of spasms "combined" or "simultaneous" seizures. Gobbi *et al.* (1987) suggested the term of *Periodic Spasms*, and supposed that a focal ictal event followed by the cluster of spasms constitutes a kind of partial seizure with secondary generalization, and this latter consisting of the spasms which repeat in periodic sequence in a more or less prolonged series, triggered by abnormal interaction between the cortex and the brainstem (Gobbi *et al.*, 1987; Gobbi *et al.*, 1996). Partial seizures sometimes may appear during the cluster (Gobbi *et al.*, 1996) and may interact with a succession of epileptic spasms in a close but variable temporal association (Pachatz *et al.*, 2003). Differently, Ohtsuka *et al.* (2001) found that the spasm-spasm interval is not influenced by the concurrent occurrence of an ictal focal event. Finally, the cluster of spasms may start without being preceded by any other seizure. The evolution of ESOWS is variable, and in the case of brain malformation, they may persist until adulthood, unchanged and resistant to AEDs (Gobbi *et al.*, 1987; Gobbi *et al.*, 1996; Pachatz *et al.*, 2003).

Figures 1 and *2* show a typical example of a cluster of spasms without any clinical and/or EEG manifestations preceding the cluster in a patient with cryptogenic epilepsy with focal adversive seizures associated with epileptic spasms. *Figures 3* and *4* show a typical example of a focal occipital seizure followed by a cluster of epileptic spasms, in an infant with perinatal anoxic-ischemic encephalopathy.

ESOWS with onset after the age of one year
(Late Onset Epileptic Spasms – LOES outside WS)

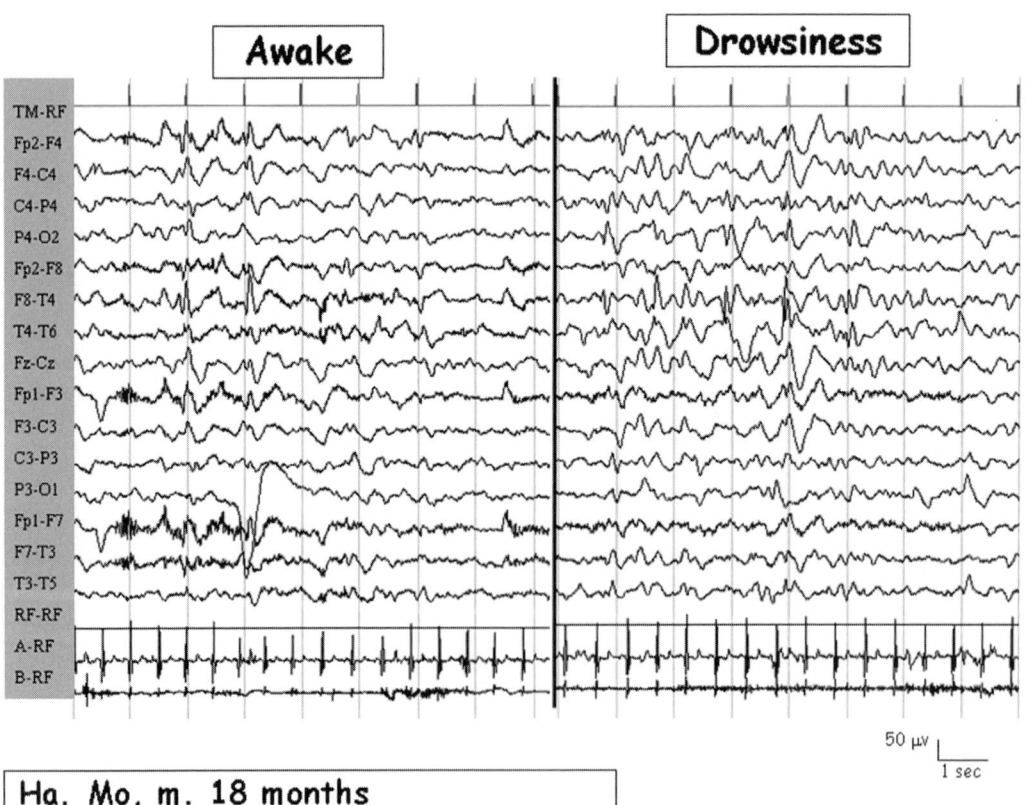

Figure 1. Patient affected by cryptogenic epilepsy with focal adversive seizures and epileptic spasms. Interictal EEG.
On the left (awake), sharp waves in the right fronto-temporal region, increased during drowsiness (on the right)

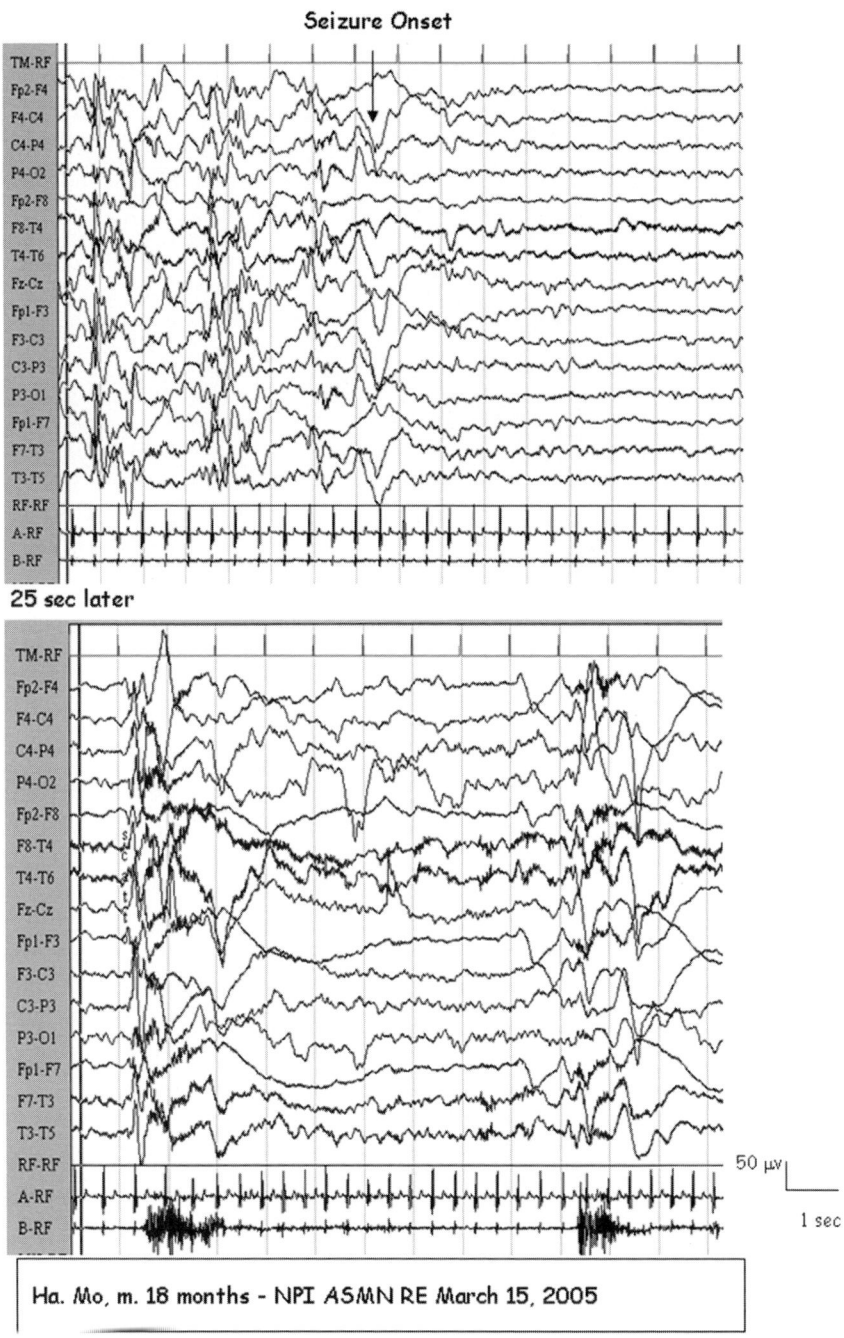

Figure 2. Same patient of figure one. Cluster of spasms without any preceding clinical and/or EEG manifestations.
Seizure starts with an electrical event consisting of high voltage slow wave with superimposed fast rhythm complex (arrow). 25 seconds later cluster of spasms concomitant with a high voltage slow wave with superimposed fast rhythm complex.

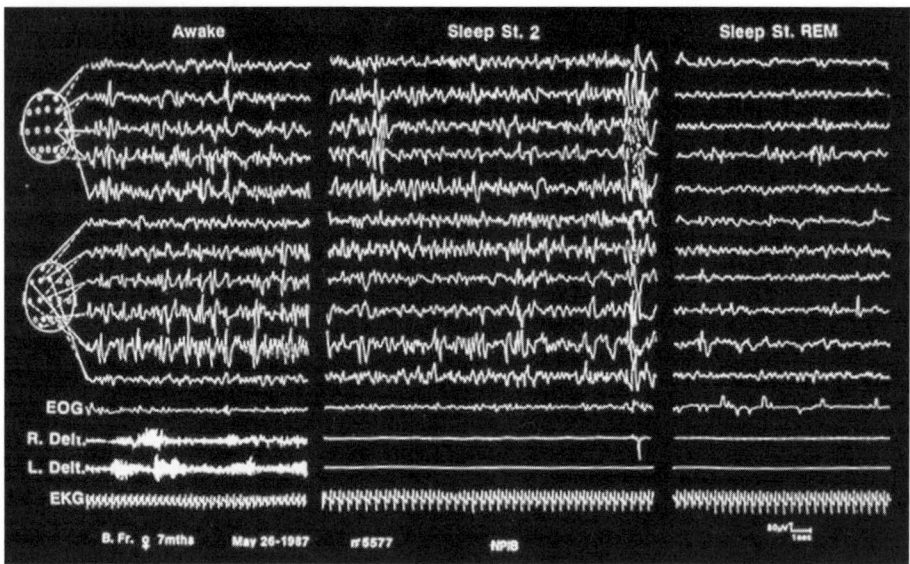

Figure 3. Infant with perinatal anoxic-ischemic encephalopathy.
Interictal EEG. Multifocal paroxysmal abnormalities predominant in the posterior areas (awake, on the left), increased by slow sleep (sleep st 2, on the middle). EEG abnormalities became more focalized again during REM sleep (on the right).

LOES outside WS in Partial Epilepsies

Amongst the seven patients reported in 1987 by Gobbi et al. the spasms started after the first year of life in some. Similar cases have been reported by Ohtsuka Y (1998), Bednarek et al. (1998), Ohtsuka et al. (2001), and Eisermann et al. (2006). The aetiology may be cryptogenic (Gobbi et al., 1987; Bednarek et al., 1998; Eisermann et al., 2006), but usually brain malformations have been detected on neuroimaging (Gobbi et al., 1996; Pini et al., 1996; Bednarek et al., 1998; Ohtsuka et al., 2001). Eisermann et al. (2006) reported that patients with cryptogenic LOES have consistent temporal or fronto-temporal EEG abnormalities instead of occipital or frontal predominance of the interictal abnormalities as respectively reported in WS and in LGS. Thus, they consider cryptogenic LOES as an intermediate condition between WS and LGS.

The evolution is poor because the spasms tend to persist unchanged during the evolution, usually resistant to AEDs or evolve into a focal or multifocal epilepsy (Gobbi et al., 1987; Eiserman et al., 2006). Cognitive and behavioural disorders have been reported in more than 2/3 of the patients, and the response to vigabatrin is worse than in IS of WS (Bednarek et al., 1998).

LOES outside WS in generalized epileptic encephalopathies

Several situations have to be considered. Epileptic spasms in WS may persist after 2-3 years of age without evolution to LGS. If hypsarrhythmia persists, this is a case of long-lasting West Syndrome (Ohtsuka Y, 1991; Mizukawa M., 1992). If hypsarrhythmia disappears, this is a case of severe focal or multifocal partial epilepsy (Otsuka et al., 1991). Epileptic spasms may persist in patients with Lennox Gastaut syndrome

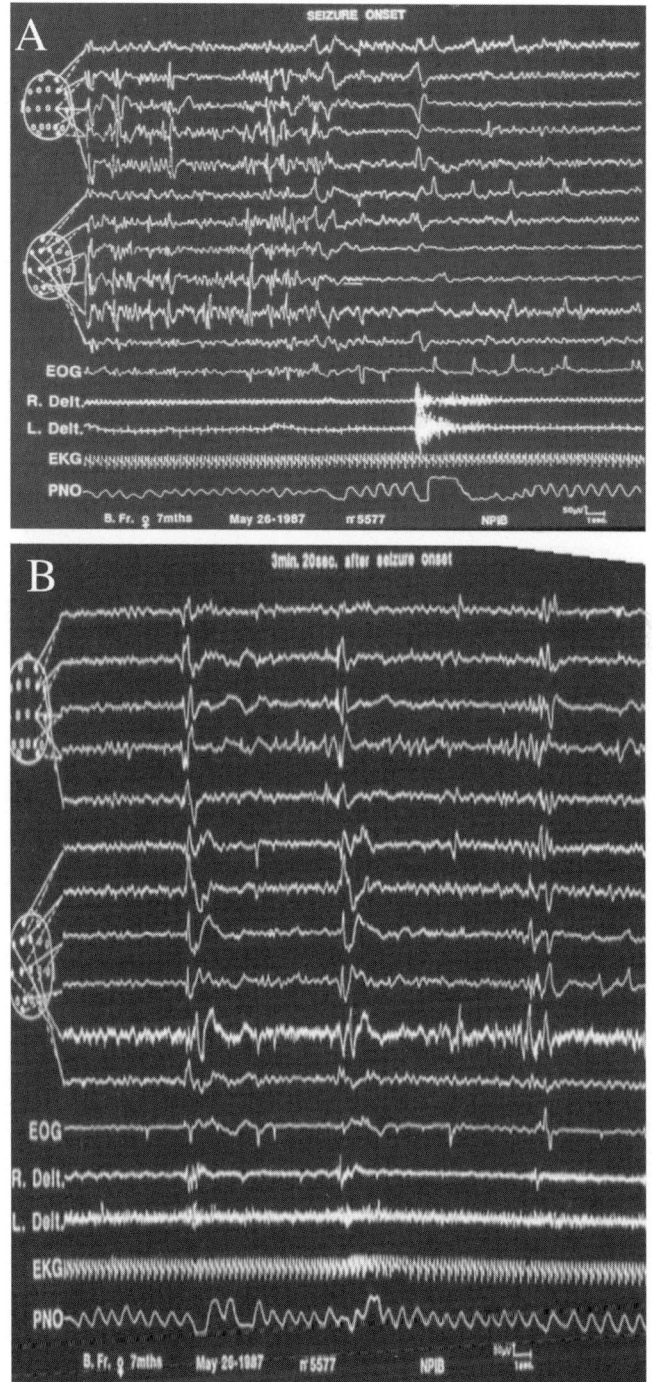

Figure 4. A. Left occipital seizure(underlined) followed by a bilateral spasm concomitant with a bilateral slow wave with superimposed fast rhythm complex.

B. Three minutes and 20 seconds later, cluster of periodic spasms.

that had evolved from WS (Shigematsu et al., 1987; Otsuka Y, 2001). In this case the frequency and the duration of the clusters is lower compared to those seen in WS. All these situations have to be included in WS. There are also rare cases of late onset epileptic spasms with typical or modified hypsarrhythmia, who have to be included in WS (Bednarek et al., 1998).

Late Onset Epileptic Spasms Outside West Syndrome have been reported in the case of cryptogenic LGS without a history of WS (Boniver et al., 1987; Donat and Wright 1991b; Ohtsuka et al., 2001). In these cases polygraphic recordings revealed that clinical and EEG characteristics of the clusters of spasms are similar to those in WS. In our personal series the cluster of spasms may be preceded by a generalized tonic seizure. These spasms have to be differentiated from tonic seizures which may be repeated in periodic sequences in patients with LGS. Lo et al. in 1991 reported children with LGS having a series of brief, repeated tonic or myoclonic seizures, in which the behavioural phenomena were more pronounced, mimicking a complex partial seizure (Lo WD, 1991). *Figure 5* shows the EEG of this peculiar seizure in a patient of our series.

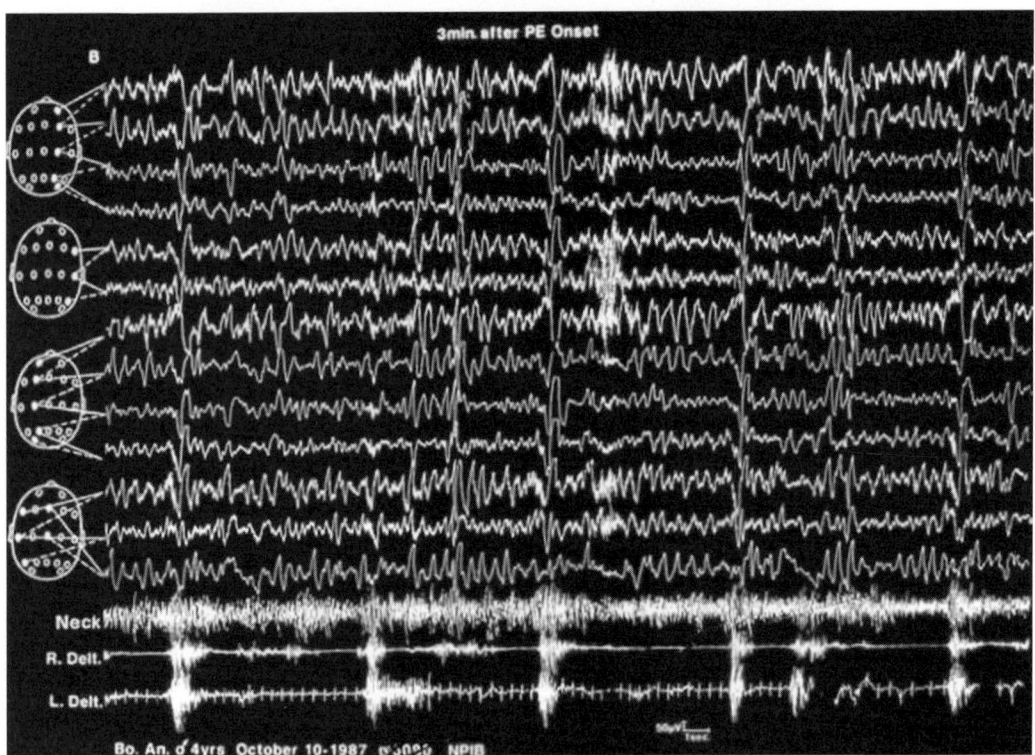

Figure 5. Children with LGS having a series of brief, repeated tonic or myoclonic seizures, in which the behavioural phenomena were more pronounced, mimicking a complex partial seizure.
Note the background slowing predominant in both frontal areas and a periodic sequence of bilateral spasms.

■ Discussion and conclusion

Spasms outside West Syndrome may be a non-epileptic or an epileptic event. Non-epileptic spasms include abdominal pain (colic), benign neonatal sleep myoclonus, hyperekplexia, Sandifer syndrome, early breath-holding spells and syncopal attacks, adverse reactions or intolerance to exogenous agents, paroxysmal dystonia and choreoathetosis (paroxysmal torticollis, benign infantile dystonia), increased Moro reflex and attacks of opisthotonus, self-gratification or masturbation-like episodes, benign paroxysmal tonic upward gaze, shuddering attacks, Fejerman syndrome (benign myoclonus of early infancy), tonic reflex seizure of early infancy (Caraballo et al., 2003), and repetitive sleep starts (Fusco et al., 1999).

Epileptic spasms outside West syndrome (ESOWS) are the spasms that do not fit the standard pattern of WS. They may start *before* the age of 1 year, but also *after* the age of one year (LOES), and may be found in the case of Cryptogenic or Lesional Partial Epilepsies and Epileptic Encephalopathies, including focal symptomatic epilepsies with neonatal, infancy and childhood onset, Early Myoclonic Encephalopathy, Ohtahara syndrome, Aicardi Syndrome, Periodic Spasms with different aetiologies, and some cases of LGS (Gobbi et al., 1987 and 1996; Ohtsuka et al., 2001). ESOWS constitute a group of seizures with an extremely heterogeneous clinical semiology, while the ictal EEG-polygraphic pattern tends to be quite stereotyped and similar to that of WS. Hypsarrhythmia has never been reported in these patients. In the case of LOES, Bednarek et al. (1998) stated that interictal EEG patterns were within the range of classically described modifications of hypsarrhythmia. This statement is in contrast with our experience, since no patient in our series had hypsarrhythmia, and it has not been confirmed by Eisermann et al. in their more recent report of 2006.

The evolution ESOWS is usually severe. Spasms usually persist unchanged during the course of the disorder, resistant to all AEDs, and concomitant with cognitive and behavioural disturbances (Gobbi et al., 1987; Bednarek et al., 1998; Ohtsuka et al., 2001). Vigabatrin is less efficacious than what is reported in West syndrome. Corticosteroids may have only transient efficacy. There is not consistent experience with ketogenic diet. In cryptogenic LOES cognitive and psychomotor deterioration occurr only after the onset of the ES, and they are usually moderate concerning language and behaviour, but may also be totally absent (Eiserman et al., 2006).

A careful clinical history and video-EEG polygraphic recordings are mandatory for diagnosis of ES and to differentiate spasms from myoclonic seizures (Bednareck et al., 1998). Patients with cryptogenic IS reported by Caraballo et al. in 2003 have to be differentiated from those with WS because of lack of hypsarrhythmia or modified hypsarrhythmia, the association with focal seizures, and resistance to the AEDs. Patients with LOES outside West syndrome differ from those with WS because of late onset of the spasms, absence of hypsarrhythmia (Gobbi et al., 1987; Bednarek et al., 1998; Eisermann et al., 2006), and a frequent tonic component of the limb contraction (Eisermann et al., 2006). LOES outside West syndrome differ from LGS because of lack of slow spike-wave activity, lack of burst of fast activity, diffuse polyspike waves and tonic seizures during sleep, and lack of atypical absences (Gobbi et al., 1987; Bednarek et al., 1998; Eisermann et al., 2006).

Eisermann et al. (2006) suggest that temporal or fronto-temporal localization of the interictal EEG abnormalities in patients with cryptogenic late onset ESOWS may account for a dysfunction of the maturation process of the temporal lobe, which explains their delayed age at onset. In fact, variability in the localization of interictal abnormalities may be related to differences in progression of the maturational process and may account for the age-relation of certain epileptic encephalopathies. Posterior areas become mature during the first year of life and that may account for the posterior predominance of spike waves in WS. Frontal lobes became mature in the first decade of life and may account for anterior predominance of interictal abnormalities in LGS. On the contrary, the maturation of temporal lobes is difficult to determine because of their heterogeneity due to major structural differences between mesial and lateral parts (Eisermann et al., 2006).

The mechanisms involved in the occurrence of ES are far to be demonstrated. It has been suggested that an abnormal functional interaction between cortex and subcortical structures may be the cause of cluster of spasms (Dulac et al., 1999; Chugani et al., 1992). Cluster of spasms preceded by an ictal focal event may correspond to a single partial seizure with a peculiar secondary generalization (the spasms), triggered by abnormal interaction between the cortex and the brainstem (Gobbi G, 1987; Gobbi G, 1996), Probably, the spasms themselves originate from subcortical structures (Ohtsuka et al., 2001).

In conclusion the epileptic spasms outside WS constitute a heterogeneous group of epileptic seizures, which may start at different ages, and which may be present in lesional or cryptogenic epilepsies. LOES outside WS may constitute a specific epileptic syndrome, partial in type (Gobbi et al., 1987) and cryptogenic in aetiology (Eisermann et al., 2006).

References

Aicardi J. The agyria-pachygyria complex: a spectrum of cortical malformations. *Brain Dev* 1991; 13: 1-8.

Aicardi J. Early myoclonic encephalopathy (neonatal myoclonic encephalopathy). In: Roger J, Bureau M, Dravet Ch, Dreifuss FE, Perret A, Wolf P, eds. *Epileptic syndromes in infancy, childhood and adolescence*, 2nd ed.. London: John Libbey, 1992: 13-23.

Bednarek N, Motte J, Soufflet C, Plouin P, Dulac O. Evidence of late onset infantile spasms. *Epilepsia* 1998; 39: 55-60.

Blume WT, Luders HO, Mizrahi E, Tassinari C, van Emde Boas W, Engel J Jr. Glossary of descriptive terminology for ictal semiology: report of the ILAE task force on classification and terminology. *Epilepsia* 2001; 42: 1212-8.

Boniver C, Dravet C, Bureau M, Roger J. Idiopathic Lennox-Gastaut syndrome. In: Wolf P, Dam M, Janz D, Dreifuss FE, eds. *Advances in epileptology*, vol. 16. New York, NY: Raven Press, 1987: 195-200.

Caraballo RH, Fejerman N, Dalla Bernardina B, Ruggieri V, Cersosimo R, Medina C et al. Epileptic spasms in clusters without hypsarrhythmia in infancy. *Epileptic Disord* 2003; 5: 109-13.

Carrazana EJ, Lombroso CT, Mikati M, Helmers S, Holmes GL. Facilitation of Infantile Spasms by Partial Seizures. *Epilepsia* 1993; 34: 97-109.

Chevrie JJ, Aicardi J. The Aicardi syndrome. In: Pedley TA, Meldrum BS, editors. *Recent advances in epilepsy, vol. 3*. Edinburgh: Churchill Livingstone, 1986: 189-10.

Chugani HT, Shewmon DA, Sankar R, Chen BC, Phelps ME. Infantile Spasms: II. Lenticular Nuclei and Brain Stem activation on Positron Emission Tomography. *Ann Neurol* 1992; 31: 212-9.

Commission on Classification and Terminology of the International League Against Epilepsy. Proposal for classification of epilepsies and epileptic syndromes. *Epilepsia* 1985; 26: 268-78.

Commission on Classification and Terminology of the International League Against Epilepsy. Proposal for revised classification of epilepsies and epileptic syndromes. *Epilepsia* 1989; 30: 389-99.

Commission on Pediatric Epilepsy of the International League Against Epilepsy. Workshop on infantile spasms. *Epilepsia* 1992; 33: 195.

Donat JF, Wright FS. Simultaneous infantile spasms and partial seizures. *J Child Neurol* 1991; 6: 246-50.

Donat JF, Wright FS. Seizures in series: similarities between seizures of the west and Lennox-Gastaut syndromes *Epilepsia*. 1991; 32: 504-9.

Dulac O, Chiron C, Robain O, Plouin P, Jambaque I, Pinard J. Infantile spasms: a pathophysiological hypothesis. In: Nehlig A, Motte J, moshé SL, Plouin P eds. *Childhood epilepsies and brain development*, London: John Libbey, 1999: 93-102.

Eisermann MM, Ville D, Soufflet C, Plouin P, Chiron C, Dulac O, *et al*. Cryptogenic late-onset epileptic spasms: an overlooked syndrome of early childhood? *Epilepsia* 2006; 47: 1035-42.

Fusco L, Vigevano F. Ictal clinical electroencephalographic findings of spasms in West syndrome. *Epilepsia* 1993; 34: 671-78.

Fusco L, Pachatz C, Cusmai R, Vigevano F. Repetitive sleep starts in neurologically impaired children: an unusual non-epileptic manifestation in otherwise epileptic subjects. *Epileptic Disord* 1999; 1: 63-7.

Gobbi G, Bruno L, Pini A, Giovanardi Rossi P, Tassinari CA. Periodic spasms: an unclassified type of epileptic seizure in childhood. *Dev Med Child Neurol* 1987; 29: 766-75.

Gobbi G, Pini A, Parmeggiani A, Santucci M, Giovanardi Rossi P, Guerrini R. Periodic spasms in cortical dysplasia. In: Guerrini R, Andermann F, Canapicchi R, Roger J, Zifkin BG, Pfanner P, eds. *Dysplasias of cerebral cortex and epilepsy*, Philadelphia, PA: Lippincott-Raven, 1996: 311-21.

Hrachovy R.A., Frost J.D. Jr. Infantile spasms: a disorder of the developing nervous system. In Kellaway P, Noebels JL eds. "Problems and concepts in developmental neurophysiology" Baltimore: The Johns Hopkins University Press 1989: 131-47.

Lo WD, Donat JF and Wright FS. Tonic and myoclonic seizures in Lennox Gastaut Syndrome mistaken as complex partial seizures. *J Epilepsy* 1991; 4: 211-5.

Lux AL, Osborne JP. A Proposal for Case Definitions and Outcome Measures in Studies of Infantile Spasms and West Syndrome: Consensus Statement of the West Delphi Group. *Epilepsia* 2004; 45: 1416-28.

Mizukawa M. Severe epilepsy with multiple independent spike foci. *Tenkankenkyu (J Jpn Epil Soc)* 1992; 10: 78-87.

Ohtahara S, Ohtsuka Y, Yamatogi Y, Oka E, Inoue H. Early-infantile epileptic encephalopathy with suppression-bursts. In: Roger J, Bureau M, Dravet Ch, Dreifuss FE, Perret A, Wolf P, eds. *Epileptic syndromes in infancy, childhood and adolescence, 2nd ed*. London: John Libbey, 1992: 25-34.

Ohtsuka Y, Amano R, Mizukawa M, Maniwa S, Ohtahara S. Longterm prognosis of the Lennox-Gastaut syndrome: consideration in its evolutional change. In: Fukuyama Y, Kamoshita S, Ohtsuka C, Suzuki Y, eds. *Modern perspectives of child neurology*, Tokyo: The Japanese Society of Child Neurology, 1991: 215-22.

Ohtsuka Y, Oka E, Terasaki T, Ohtahara S. Aicardi syndrome: a longitudinal clinical and electroencephalographic study. *Epilepsia* 1993; 34: 627-34.

Ohtsuka Y, Murashima I, Asano T, Oka E, Ohtahara S. Partial seizures in West Syndrome. *Epilepsia* 1996; 37: 1060-7.

Ohtsuka Y. West syndrome and its related epileptic syndromes. *Epilepsia* 1998; 39 (suppl 5): 30-7.

Ohtsuka Y, Ohno S, Oka E. Electroclinical characteristics of hemimegalencephaly. *Pediatr Neurol* 1999; 20: 390-3.

Ohtsuka Y, Kobayashi K, Ogino T, Oka E. Spasms in clusters in epilepsies other than typical West syndrome. *Brain Dev* 2001 23: 473-81.

Pachatz C, Fusco L, Vigevano F. Epileptic spasms and partial seizures as a single ictal event. *Epilepsia.* 2003; 44: 693-700.

Pini A, Merlini L, Tome FM, Chevallay M, Gobbi G. Merosin-negative congenital muscular dystrophy, occipital epilepsy with periodic spasms and focal cortical dysplasia. Report of three Italian cases in two families. *Brain Dev* 1996; 18: 316-22.

Shigematsu H, Yagi K, Seino M. A peculiar minor seizures characterized by flexor spasms in Lennox-Gastaut syndrome evolved from West syndrome. *Jpn J Psychiatr Neurol* 1987; 41: 457-8.

Vigevano F, Fusco L, Granata T, Fariello G, Di Rocco C, Cusmai R. Hemimegalencephaly: clinical and EEG characteristics. In: Guerrini R, Andermann F, Canapicchi R, Roger J, Zifkin BG, Pfanner P, eds. *Dysplasias of cerebral cortex and epilepsy*, Philadelphia, PA: Lippincott-Raven, 1996: 285-94.

Wirrell E, Tong K. Pachygyria associated with childhood-onset epileptic spasms. *J Child Neurol* 1998; 13: 461-4.

Yamamoto N, Watanabe K, Negro T et al. Partial seizures evolving to infantile spasms. *Epilepsia* 1988; 29: 31-40.

New paediatric behavioural and electrophysiological tests of brain function for vision and attention to predict cognitive and neurological outcomes

Janette Atkinson

*Visual Development Unit, University College London
& University of Oxford*

Impairments of visual function have been demonstrated in West syndrome, although the brain basis of these deficits is not completely understood (*e.g.* Guzzetta *et al.*, 2002; Randò *et al.*, 2004; Randò *et al.*, 2005; Baranello *et al.*, 2006). These effects are not surprising given that in the adult brain over half of the neural circuitry is involved in some aspect of visual processing. As visual function develops considerably over the first year of life and this is often the time when West syndrome is first diagnosed, we might expect that brain plasticity in this early period sets the limits for recovery from infantile seizures. It is precisely this plasticity which we must understand if we are to give effective early treatment and the rationale behind our research is to try to measure specific deficits and relate them to the underlying brain mechanisms.

In this chapter I will discuss current theories of visual development which have been developed from results using new tests to measure functioning in specific areas and neural systems. Hopefully this may throw light on the underlying processing deficits in infants and children with developmental disorders, such as West syndrome.

For more than twenty years the team of the Visual Development Unit, funded by the Medical Research Council and three Universities (Cambridge, University College London and Oxford) has used a neurobiological approach to devise theories and measures of both normal and abnormal eye-brain development and neural plasticity from birth to adulthood. We have developed safe, reliable methods of assessment over the entire range of visual abilities from children with multiple disabilities and severe problems such as "cortical blindness", specific visual problems such as strabismus, amblyopia and refractive error, perceptual and visucognitive problems and children with developmental disorders such as Williams syndrome, autism and dyspraxia (*e.g.* see reviews Atkinson 1989, 1991, Atkinson and Van Hof-van Duin, 1993; Atkinson 2000 and papers Smith *et al.*, 1989; Atkinson *et al.*, 2002a; Mercuri *et al.*, 1997c; Atkinson *et al.*, 2001; Atkinson *et al.*, 2003b; Spencer *et al.*, 2000; O'Brien *et al.*, 2002). Early visual tests have proved to be prognostic indicators of neurological progress, and predict cognitive and neurological outcome in later years (*e.g.* Mercuri *et al.*, 1998b; Mercuri *et al.*, 2004; Atkinson, 2003). For this reason they are sometimes called "early surrogate outcome measures". We are currently using such measures to gauge the success of intervention and rehabilitation in clinical trials for infant populations, such as for infants born very prematurely before 32 weeks gestation, who are at high risk of early brain damage.

For many years we have collaborated with neonatologists and paediatric neurologists, first in Addenbrookes Hospital (Cambridge), then Stella Maris and CNR (Pisa), Catholic University in Rome, Pavia and the Hammersmith Hospital (London). We assess visual brain function both through behavioural and electrophysiological tests we have devised, comparing our results to results from standard and new brain imaging techniques. The clinical groups have included children with cerebral palsy (*e.g.* Atkinson, 1989; Atkinson & Van Hof-van-Duin, 1993), infants with HIE (Mercuri *et al.*, 1996; Mercuri *et al.*, 1997a; Mercuri *et al.*, 1997b; King, 1997) infants with focal infarcts (Hood *et al.*, 1989; Hood & Atkinson, 1990b; Atkinson & Hood, 1994; Mercuri *et al.*, 1995; Mercuri *et al.*, 1996; Mercuri *et al.*, 1998a; Biagioni *et al.*, 2002; Mercuri *et al.*, 2003) infants who have undergone hemispherectomy to relieve intractable epilepsy (Braddick *et al.*, 1992; Morrone *et al.*, 1999) and children who have been born very prematurely (*e.g.* Atkinson *et al.*, 1990; Atkinson *et al.*, 1991; Atkinson, 2002; Atkinson *et al.*, 2002c; Atkinson, 2003; Atkinson *et al.*, 2003a; Atkinson *et al.*, 2004).

The chapter is in several sections:

– Models of normal visual development.

– Measures for gauging onset of functioning in the cortex.

– Tests for measuring the development of the "dorsal" and "ventral" cortical streams: ABCDEFV (Atkinson Battery of Child Development for Examining Functional Vision); Tests of Frontal Lobe function and executive control of attention:

■ Model of normal visual development

A schematic of our current neurobiological model of normal visual development in infancy is shown in *Figure 1*, together with a schematic diagram of different modules within the dorsal stream. A brief description of this model is necessary so that the reader understands the rationale behind specific tests. A description of the model can be found in several published papers and chapters (Atkinson, 1984; Braddick *et al.*, 1989; Atkinson, 1998; Atkinson & Braddick, 2003), with a full description in Atkinson (2000). At the top of the figure we show the state of the newborn visual system at birth. Moving down the vertical age line the cortex starts to become functional, with different cortical modules having different onset times and attentional mechanisms for controlling eye and head movements start to operate. These are first

New paediatric behavioural and electrophysiological tests of brain function

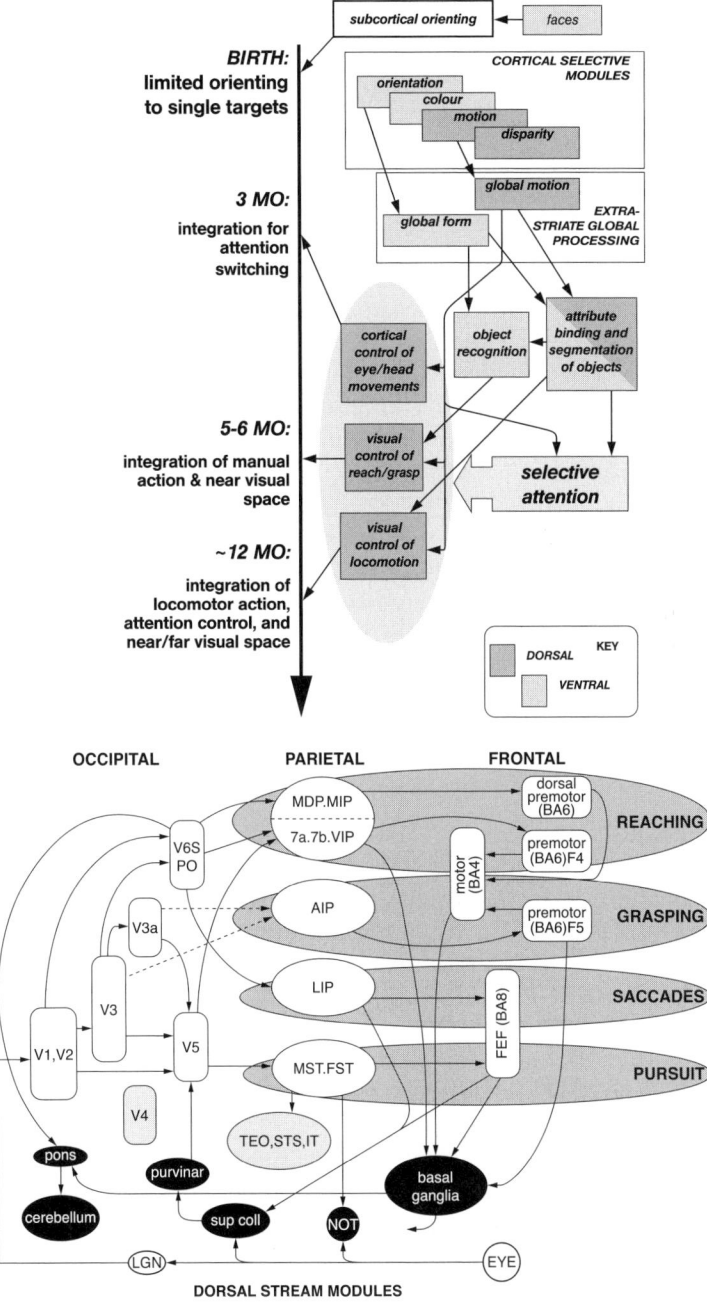

Figure 1.

Above is a schematic of the Atkinson and Braddick model of early visual development. The dorsal and ventral streams are coded differently.

Below is a schematic of Atkinson's model of modules within the dorsal stream. These are for controlling reaching, grasping, saccadic eye movements and pursuit eye movements. This is for an adult visual system subcortically controlled and after 3 months come under cortical control. In the figure the modules are divided into those which are thought to be part of the ventral stream (orientation, colour, face recognition) and those part of the dorsal stream (motion, binocularity, attention and actions including voluntary eye movements). These systems are discussed further below.

■ Newborn vision

Eye movements and orienting. The newborn infant starts life with a well developed subcortical visual system, allowing saccadic tracking and orienting to salient stimuli in the periphery, mainly under the control of circuitry in the midbrain including the superior colliculus. There is evidence for subcortical control in newborns of the visual optokinetic responses (OKN) for both directions of movement (optokinetic eye movements for pattern movement to left and right with binocular viewing by the newborn). In newborns there is an asymmetry in the OKN response when the child views monocularly favouring OKN responses for nasalward pattern movement, demonstrating a functioning crossed subcortical pathway via the nucleus of the optic tract. The OKN cortical response, underpinning eye movements in a temporalward direction (away from the nose) for monocular viewing, is not seen until 3-4 months after birth. Infants with early hemispherectomy show evidence for subcortical control in early life of the visual optokinetic responses for both directions of movement (OKN for pattern movement to left and right). However, after about 5 months of age the direction which would normally involve control from the damaged hemisphere becomes non-functional despite the intact subcortical system (Braddick et al., 1992; Morrone et al., 1999).

One interesting finding concerning newborn vision is the apparent sensitivity to schematic face-like stimuli- "the three symmetrically arranged blobs" stimulus representing the eyes and mouth (for reviews see Morton & Johnson, 1991; de Haan et al., 2002; de Haan et al., 2003). The underpinning neural processing for this is unknown but processing within the pulvinar has been suggested. A second suggestion is that it represents an upper visual field bias in newborn perception rather than a true cortical response (Turati et al., 2002).

■ Visual development over the first six months of life

Perception of pattern, colour, movement and depth: Neurons in the subcortical visual system are not sensitive to changes of orientation, colour, directional movement or disparity. Detection and discrimination of these visual attributes depends on sensitivity in particular populations of neurons in the striate visual cortex (V1) and extrastriate cortex (*e.g.* V2, V3, V3A, V4, V5) We have shown that for the visual cortical modules subserving the perception of orientation of lines (or slant), direction of movement, binocular correlation and binocular disparity and colour discrimination, each module has its own functional time course for development, within the first few months of life for normal development. Orientation and colour discrimination can be demonstrated in newborns in the first few weeks of life, but these discrimination systems becomes more finely tuned, both spatially and temporally over the first

12 months of life. Discrimination of direction of movement can be demonstrated in infants over 2 months of age (e.g. Wattam-Bell 1991). Binocular correlation and disparity discrimination (stereopsis-3D vision) can be demonstrated from 4 months post term age upwards in normally developing infants and sensitivity to binocular disparity increases with age (e.g. Braddick et al., 1980, Braddick et al., 1983).

■ Development for mechanisms of selective visual attention

Many visual tasks require a selective control process which determines the relevant spatial region, the goal of a visually directed action, or the required mode of processing. The development of such attentional control processes is an important part of visual development, and one that is frequently disordered in developmental pathology. The most basic form of selection is the selection of a target for fixation, in the face of competing targets, a system believed to involve parietal/occipital circuits, with connections to frontal eye fields and the superior colliculus. We have studied how this process, requiring disengagement from current fixation, develops after birth and have gathered extensive normative data.

To measure this we developed the fixation shift paradigm for examining the ability of infants to make saccadic shifts of attention from a foveated target to one in left or right peripheral field (Atkinson & Braddick 1985; Atkinson et al., 1988; Atkinson et al., 1992). This test reveals that normal infants under 3-4 months show difficulties of disengaging from the central target under conditions where the central and peripheral targets simultaneously compete for attention. This "sticky fixation" persists in some older children with cortical and/or basal ganglia lesions (Atkinson et al., 1993; Mercuri et al., 1996; Mercuri et al., 1997a). This test provides an indicator of the maturation, and asymmetries, of cortical mechanisms controlling the disengagement and shift of attention. It is likely to be related to hemianopia often seen alongside "neglect" in adult stroke patients.

■ Development of dorsal and ventral streams

The dorsal and ventral streams are represented as separate in the developmental model in *Figure 1* although in practice they operate in a coordinated fashion in everyday perception. There are several reviews of our studies on dorsal and ventral stream development (for example, Atkinson 2000; Atkinson & Braddick 2003; Braddick et al., 2003) and so only a brief description will be given here.

The starting point for our theoretical model of visual development in areas beyond primary visual cortex (V1) is based largely on electrophysiological studies of non-human primates and studies of adult neurological patients with focal lesions in parietal, temporal and frontal cortex. From non-human primate studies cortical neurones have been identified, specific for particular visual attributes and clustered in anatomically distinct areas. Areas were defined selective for motion information (V5 or MT) and colour (V4) (Zeki 1974, 1978, 1983a, 1983b, 1993; Maunsell & Van Essen 1983a, 1983b, 1987). These theories postulated that both visual "where?" and "what?"

responses were largely under cortical control, with the tectal loops being regarded as largely superseded substations for "reflex" actions. Ungerleider and Mishkin (1982) suggested that the two streams are associated with different visual capacities. There is a largely parietal mechanism involved in localizing objects within a spatial array and intimately linked to eye movement mechanisms of selective attention, and temporal lobe mechanisms tuned to "what" aspects such as form, colour and face recognition. Clinical observations of patients with specific focal lesions support this dissociation between loss of position or movement perception and deficits of object recognition in particular patients (e.g. Damasio & Benton 1979; Zihl et al., 1983; Milner and Goodale, 1994). A second model was proposed for the adult visual system based on the idea of two anatomically distinct streams, the parvocellular and magnocellular streams. The two streams are distinct morphologically at ganglion cell and LGN levels, project to different parts of primary visual cortex, V1, and continue within independent cortical streams to V4 and V5 (Maunsell & Van Essen 1983a, 1983b; Maunsell & Newsome 1987; Livingstone & Hubel 1988). The parvocellular based system has been proposed to subserve detailed form vision and colour while the magnocellular system subserves movement perception and some aspects of stereoscopic vision. Mausell and Van Essen (1983a, 1983b) popularized the easily remembered name, MT, for the medial temporal area (equivalent to V5) for the "movement" specific stream as opposed to the "form" and "colour" stream via V2 and V4. There has been the suggestion that the divide between "where?" and "what?" systems in the cortex is a result of the the initial division between different cell types of the parvocellular and magnocellular systems. We have looked at the time course of development of specific cortical modules in infant development. There is some evidence to suggest that parvocellular – based systems may become operational slightly earlier than magnocellular systems and that the two systems are not synchronized in early development (Atkinson, 1992).

Our current models take as their basis the distinction made by Goodale and Milner (1995) between the dorsal "where" and ventral "what" cortical streams. This is that there is not only separate coding within the streams of different visual attributes or stimulus properties, such as colour and movement, but rather there are two broad categories of visual coding. One stream is useful for perceptual processing (ventral) and one for controlling actions (dorsal). As the ventral pathways contain specialized areas for face perception and the dorsal stream contains systems for controlling eye movements, reaching and grasping, we can rename these systems the "who?" and the "how?" systems. One system helps us decide what and who we are looking at and one system decides the appropriate responses and actions to be made on these objects. Rather than two distinct streams, Goodale and Milner suggest multiple modules, loosely connected into two broad streams of processing, with each operating in an internal coordinated fashion. The relatively fast "action" stream has a very short memory and is for automatic "unconscious" immediate responses, whereas the ventral stream controls "conscious" awareness and interactions with more long lasting elaborate memory stores.

When this model is applied to human development we can see that it is not only possible to have differential timing of functional development between the two major cortical streams, but is also possible to have differential development, internally, within different modules within each stream. In infants, the multiple "action" modules within the dorsal stream, controlling head, eyes, arm, hand and general body movements each show their own developmental timecourse (see *Figure 1* for a schematic of these different parts of the dorsal stream). The first action module to become functional is the one used for making exploratory eye movements and for shifting attention through head and eye movements from one object to another seemingly "at will". The substrate for these head and eye movements are already operational at birth but change and improve dramatically in the first few months of life. This is followed in development by functioning in the action module controlling exploratory "reaching" and "grasping". Next the action module controlling independent walking starts to function. Of course early functioning in each of these action modules is not adult-like. It can take months or years for these systems to be identical to the adult brain modules. All these action programmes must involve some spatial analysis of the visual layout, but there may be quite different scales within spatial representations used for different systems. For example for reaching and grasping the infant only needs a spatial representation of space which is relatively near to the body. However, this space may need to be extended if the child starts to use tools to extend the spatial area of control of the hands in order to manipulate objects at a distance. It is well known that relatively young infants, of a few months, can learn to operate a string that is attached to a mobile so that when the string is moved the mobile moves. This means that the infant's understanding of indirect causality is already present and the movements made near to the body (moving the string) is already associated with bringing about actions in more distant space. We do not know from these studies to what extent we can stretch the distance between the hand and the mobile and still have correlated behaviour. For independent walking both peripheral vision and spatial layout some distance from the child must be represented to enable the child to find objects in spatial locations that are further away than arm's length. We know there are limitations to this understanding; however, from primate studies it seems likely that some initial perceptual analysis will be common to visual exploration, manual exploration and locomotive exploration. We might imagine that the very early stages of visual analysis involve common pathways to VI and early parts of the ventral stream, with the integration of this information from the dorsal stream. The appropriate motor programmes and fuller spatial representations in the dorsal stream follow this early processing. It may be that for different action modules it is this integration which is delayed. Alternatively, we might consider that the spatial representations for modules which develop later are in some way more complex or involve integration over numerous subsystems for them to be effective. This is certainly true when we compare the reaching and grasping module with the one for independent walking. Vestibular and peripheral optic flow information must be integrated with elaborate coordinated leg movements, together with mechanisms for analysing depth and distance in central field, for successful walking to a target. However, for reaching and grasping the peripheral optic flow information and vestibular information can be largely ignored while using depth and distance information in nearby space. For reaching and grasping, a spatial representation of the general nearby layout of objects will enable successful retrieval of objects, whereas both a detailed depth and distance map and a larger scale spatial map of objects around the room will be necessary for a child to locomote to one part of space and retrieve the object *i.e.* locate, travel to, reach and grasp, in sequence. However, it is difficult to think of visual saccadic exploration and selection of visual targets using scaled representations of depth and distance, as being "simple" in any sense. Once again the same depth and distance cues must be correctly interpreted to gauge the correct position and distance for the object to be focussed on the retina and the eye movements to foveate an object, when shifting attention from one object to another, must be precise if they are to yield useful information. Eye movement control systems are extremely complex and it is difficult to understand why, in terms of ecological validity, the infant in the first months of life has such an elaborate system functioning very similarly in terms of temporal parameters to the mature system in the adult, with relatively little visual input or learning being necessary to develop this system.

As well as these overt action systems, there must be internal covert systems of attention and memory. Here an imaginary line has been drawn between visual cortical modules for decoding incoming sensory and perceptual information and areas for categorising and storing this information in visual memory buffers. This line is sometimes drawn between "perception" and "cognition". However, the more we take on a neurobiological approach and consider the anatomical and functional connections and interactions between different modules, the more difficult it becomes to continue to make these distinctions. It is particularly in the area of visual attention that these boundaries are likely to be most imaginary.

■ Measures for gauging onset of functioning in the cortex

We have developed sensitive measures for infants in the first few months of life, to gauge the age of onset of function in the visual cortex. One is an electrophysiological measure and is for orientation discrimination, the basis of pattern, shape and object recognition. This is called the **"OR-VEP/VERP"** (Orientation-reversal visual evoked potential/visual event related potential) (first reference Braddick *et al.*, 1986). The second is a measure of visual attention called the **"fixation shift" paradigm (FS)** – this measures the abilities of the infant to shift visual attention from one target (or object) to another, when two targets are competing for the child's attention These tests and results from the premature cohort (see below) are shown in *Figure 2*. Both tests can be used to study children longitudinally with West Syndrome, although the electrophysiological measures become harder to interpret if the child is having continuous seizures at the time of testing.

■ Electrophysiological measures VEP/VERP

The table below gives a summary of the different stimulus parameters which can be used in electrophysiological testing to separate out different subcortical and cortical networks. The standard flash VEP usually gives a large signal/noise ratio but cannot be interpreted as a measure of cortical function. A child with severe cortical damage may still give a good VEP to a flash stroboscopic stimulus so long as signal from the

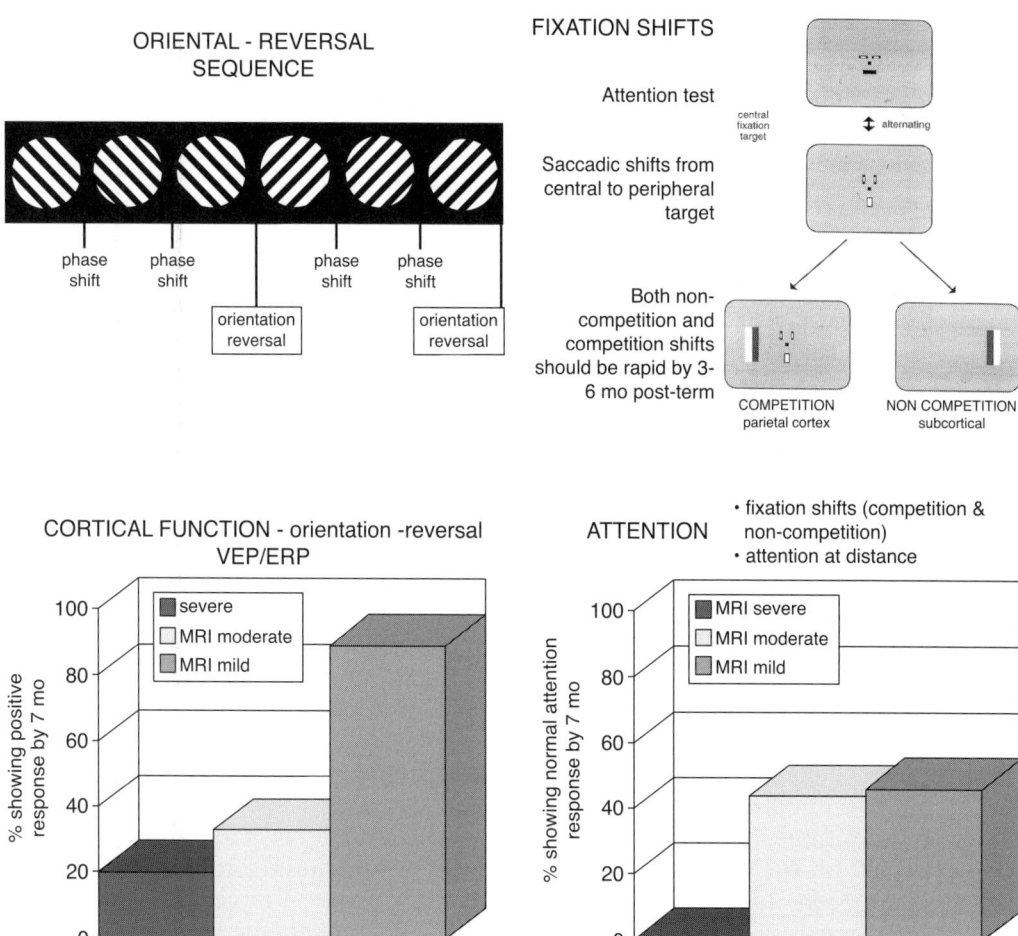

Figure 2.
Top left: schematic diagram of the stimulus sequence used for the steady state orientation reversal VEP/VERP. This change can be at 8 or 4 reversals per second
Bottom left: Division of the MRI neonatal brain imaging into three groups of premature infants – those with severe abnormalities, those with moderate and those with mild.
There is a good correlation between the brain imaging category and infants in that group showing a positive orientation reversal VEP response, at 8 reversals per second, by 7 post-term months of age.
Top right: schematic diagram of stimulus configuration used in the fixation shift paradigm, under two experimental conditions "non competition" and "competition".
Bottom right: % of premature infants showing the normal responses by 7 months of post term age relative to the category of brain abnormality seen on neonatal MRI.

retina to the brain is reasonably intact. A pattern of stripes, reversing in contrast will again give a significant response with only a subcortical system operating. However, as cortical neurones are tuned to different orientations a VEP response, timelocked to a change in orientation, indicates basic cortical processing and functioning. This is the orientation reversal stimulus in the table below.

Stimulus	Process indicated	Age of onset
flash	light response – subcortical	preterm
pattern reversal	spatial contrast response – input to cortex – not necessarily cortical	late preterm/term
orientation reversal	basic cortical pattern processing – cortical	~ 1-3 months (frequency dependent)
direction reversal	basic cortical motion processing	~ 2-3 months
global form & motion	higher level integration – extrastriate cortical mechanisms	later than 2 mo, motion before form

■ Fixation shifts

The **"fixation shifts"** test is particularly useful for measuring attentional deficits in many clinical groups. By comparing responses in the two conditions – "non-competition" (the central fixation target disappears at the same time as the peripheral laterally positioned target appears) and "competition" (the central target remains visible when the peripheral target appears) we can find whether a child is able to switch attention at will, disengaging attention from one target and switching to another Part of our evidence for these selective attentional mechanisms, controlling disengagement from one object to another when both objects are visible, being cortical rather than subcortical, comes from studies of fixation shifts in children who have undergone early hemispherectomy (Braddick et al., 1992, Atkinson and Hood, 1997). In these children there is a lack of the fixation shift response (attention shift) under "competition" on their "bad" side of space, but a normal rapid response under "competition" on the side of space opposite to the functioning cortex. When only one object appears in the periphery and the central fixation target disappears from view ("non-competition" condition) the child who has undergone hemispherectomy, but has normal subcortical areas on both sides of the brain, can shift saccadic fixation to a target on both the "good" and "bad" sides i.e. to left peripheral field and right peripheral field when fixating centrally initially.

■ Use of these cortical measures

We originally applied these cortical measures, the **orientation-reversal visual evoked potentials (OR-VEP)** and attention measures of **fixation shifts under competition** to a number of high risk groups, including: children with cerebral palsy and other neurodevelopmental disorders and known or suspected visual impairment; a cohort of very low birthweight premature infants recruited in Addenbrooke's Hospital Cambridge (Atkinson et al., 1994b); children with hemispherectomy and other unilateral lesions (Braddick et al., 1992; Morrone et al., 1999).

We followed this series of studies by the systematic longitudinal investigation of children born in the Hammersmith Hospital, with focal cerebral lesions or hypoxic-ischaemic encephalopathy, well characterised by neonatal serial MRI brain imaging and neurological examination by the neonatal and paediatric teams in the

Hammersmith. Results from these cohorts have shown that visual performance in the first months of life is a highly sensitive indicator of neurological status and outcome, but that poor visual outcome is not necessarily most strongly associated with specific damage to classically "visual" areas of the brain. Specifically, our studies found that:

a) The extent and localization of the lesion in infants with focal infarcts is not always well related to the severity of early visual impairments (Atkinson & Mercuri 1995; Mercuri et al., 1995). This suggests that early focal lesions, involving occipital structures in the visual pathways can, to some extent, be compensated for in the immature developing brain.

b) Generalised lesions in HIE, involving a number of areas of the cortex, tended to be more frequently associated with abnormal visual function (Mercuri et al., 1997a; Mercuri et al., 1999). However, normal visual function was found in infants who showed early oedema followed by a normal MRI scan after the end of the first week of life.

c) Lesions in the basal ganglia were generally associated with a more severe visual outcome, supporting the idea that certain circuits between subcortical areas and cortical areas are essential for normal visual development. All 6 children with isolated lesions of the basal ganglia showed visual deficits. This also suggests that there is little plasticity of recovery in these circuits involving the basal ganglia and that other areas cannot easily be substituted (Mercuri et al., 1997a; Atkinson et al., 1998). However, the extent to which basal ganglia damage is associated with damage to other structures, less visible on MRI, needs to be further investigated.

d) In a comparison of orientation reversal (OR) and phase reversal (PH) VEPs, as indicators of cortical function in 46 full term infants with brain lesions on MRI, we found that 50% of our cohort did not have a significant cortical OR VEP at 5 months of age. (This response would normally be expected between 3 and 5 months of age for the 8 reversals/sec stimulus and slightly earlier for 4 reversals/sec). 14% of the cohort showed continuing delayed onset of cortical function using this indicator at between 6 and 12 months of age. In 34% the VEP responses were always abnormal. Infants with focal infarction or haemorrhage on MRI tended to show normal or only mildly delayed responses, while Grade 2 or 3 HIE tended to be associated with persistent abnormalities of VEP responses (in some cases including the more robust phase-reversal response). As with other visual indicators, abnormal VEP responses were not necessarily associated with lesions seen on MRI to classical visual areas (optic radiations and occipital cortex), but were generally present if there was the concomitant involvement of basal ganglia damage. Early VEP responses, as well as being sensitive to neurological status, are a strong prognostic indicator: normal OR VEPs are reliably associated with a gross normal visual and neurodevelopmental outcome in early life, abnormal OR VEPs at 5 months of age are consistently associated with abnormal outcome (Mercuri et al., 1998a). In this group of 46 at-risk term infants, 96% of those who had shown 8 Hz OR-VEP by 5 months were neurologically normal at 3 years, compared with 57% of those who attained the response by 12 months and 0% of those in whom it was still absent at 18 months (Mercuri et al., 1998a).

We found that in group of 29 term infants with HIE, children who showed more than 3 out of 5 failures on vision tests at 5 months (optokinetic nystagmus, acuity, visual fields, fixation shifts, OR VEPs) were very likely to fail on items in ABCDEFV (see below), the structured neurological evaluation and Griffiths developmental assessment at 2 years. Children with 3 or fewer early failures were likely to have developmental quotients in the normal range at 2 years. Abnormal OKN and acuity was always associated with abnormal outcome whereas normal VEP and fixation shift was associated with normal outcome (Mercuri et al., 1998a).

OR-VEP and fixation shift testing of this group of 29 such infants gave the following results in prediction of Griffiths Developmental Quotient < 80 at 2 years:

Cortical vision test at 5 mo	Sensitivity	Specificity	Positive predictive value	Negative predictive value
fixation shift	100	59	47	100
OR-VEP	100	79	63	100

In more recent studies we have pursued this approach, including a follow up of a wide range of visual cognitive, and motor measures, in cohorts of children born very prematurely before 32 weeks who had received neonatal and term MRI at the Hammersmith Hospital.

In the first cohort study of 43 infants born before 32 weeks gestation (Atkinson 2003; Braddick et al., 2003) the protocol included at 2-6 mo post term age orientation reversal (OR) and phase reversal (PR) VEP (OR/VEP & PH VEP) fixation shifts, and core vision testing from the ABCDEFV (described below). Beyond 6 months post term age the protocol included further tests from the ABCDEFV, preschool tests of attention including tests of frontal lobe executive function (see below Russell detour box, Diamond Day/Night, counter-pointing). All tests were selected to assess particular cortical and subcortical networks, and determine whether these measures were successful in correlation with early brain damage and prediction of later outcome.

Diffuse excessive high signal intensity (DEHSI) is a common feature of the white matter in very premature infants when scanned around term, although it cannot be readily identified earlier or after about 3 months post term. The presence and degree of white matter damage (DEHSI or PVL) was classified as mild, moderate and severe depending on the extent and intensity of areas visualized with DEHSI. Some children with a diagnosis of cystic PVL were included in the group classified as severe DEHSI. Analysis shows that there is:
– a good correlation between the classification of DEHSI and all visual measures, in terms of normal or abnormal responses (against norms for gestational age) (see Figures 2 and 3);
– the severe DEHSI group (including 5 children with cystic PVL) fail on over 80% of follow-up tests;
– on the tests of spatial cognition in the ABCDEFV battery, fixation shift attention tests at 3-7 months, and the frontal preschool tests of attention, there is a high failure rate across the whole group, with less than 50% of even the "mild DEHSI" group showing normal responses for gestational age (see Figure 3);

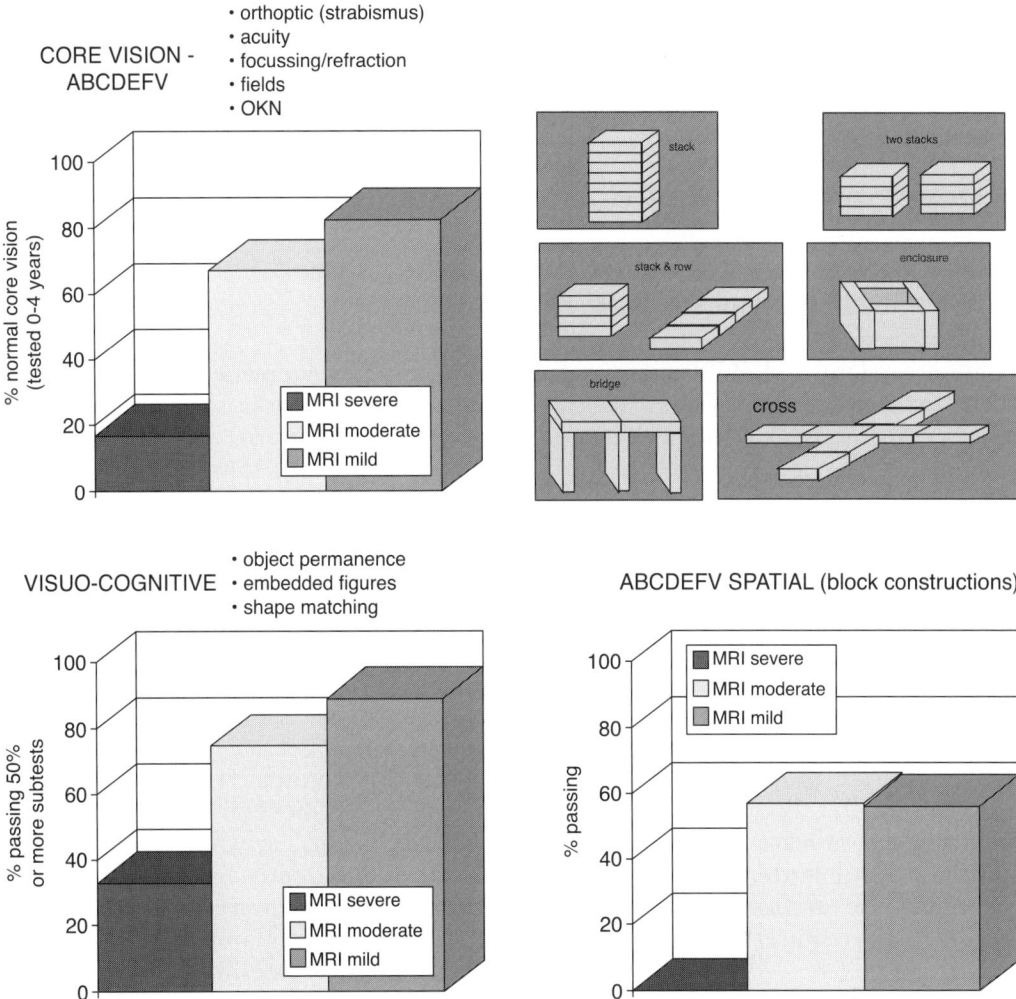

Figure 3.
Top right: three categories of premature infants with mild, moderate or severe brain damage on MRI, plotted against core vision test scores on ABCDEFV.
Bottom left: same three categories plotted against visual cognitive tests from the ABCDEFV.
Top right: different block constructions used for copying in ABCDEFV.
Bottom left: same three categories of premature infants plotted against block design copying scores from ABCDEFV.

— it appears that the early orientation-reversal VEP measure and fixation shifts paradigm may serve as early surrogate outcome measures for neurological and cognitive status at 2.5 years and possibly into the early school years. OR-VEP and fixation shift testing of this group of 24 such infants gave the following results in prediction of Griffiths Developmental Quotient < 80 at 2 years:

Cortical vision test at 5 mo	Sensitivity	Specificity	Positive predictive value	Negative predictive value
fixation shift	100	67	58	100
OR-VEP	86	65	50	92

■ Development of the dorsal and ventral cortical streams

Tests for measuring the development of the "dorsal" and "ventral" cortical streams

These are infant and child tests for gauging relative development and abnormality in the two cortical "dorsal" and "ventral" visual streams – in order to examine "dorsal stream vulnerability", using new measures of global form (pattern) and motion coherence with behavioural and electrophysiological (VEP/VERP) tests.

Global motion processing

Studies of motion psychophysics and physiology have distinguished between local motion processing – the sensitivity to direction in a small region of the image, such as a short segment of contour, and global motion processing, which allows the representation of motion over extended regions that may correspond to surfaces and objects (Braddick & Qian, 2000). The latter is usually identified with the integrative properties of V5 neurons, while the former reflects, at least in part, the smaller directional receptive fields seen in V1. Several aspects of infant performance indicate that global processes operate at an early stage of development. In a dot pattern containing a proportion of randomly moving dots, processing of the motion of individual dots cannot yield the overall direction of motion; this requires integration of motion signals over many dots, a process which can be assessed in terms of the motion coherence threshold (Newsome & Paré, 1988). Such thresholds can be measured in the preferential looking for the shearing display, and show a marked improvement over the weeks following the age at which direction discrimination first emerges (Wattam-Bell, 1994). Indeed, it could be argued that the detection of the shearing even at 100% coherence requires a kind of global operation. A related test, in which coherence is varied by changing the spread of motion directions about the mean value, shows that infants of 12 weeks and over can make direction discriminations that require integration of directional distributions whose standard deviation is up to 68 degrees (Banton et al., 1999). These results suggest that very soon after local motion signals are first available in the developing brain, the processes which integrate them into global representations are operating quite efficiently. It may be that the connectivity between V1 and extrastriate areas including V5, on which this integration is based, exists early at least in a crude form, awaiting the organization of local directional selectivity in V1 – perhaps because the latter requires some minimum level of temporal performance in the developing visual pathway before it can function.

Global motion processing compared to global form processing

The development of global motion processing – a function of extrastriate dorsal stream processing – can be compared with global processing in the ventral-stream domain of form. We have devised a measure analogous to motion coherence thresholds: subjects must detect the organization of short line segments into concentric circles, with "noise" introduced by randomizing the orientation of a proportion of the line segments (see stimulus in *Figure 4*). Neurons responding to concentric organization of this kind have been reported in area V4 in macaques (Gallant et al., 1993) – an extrastriate area occupying a similar position in the ventral stream to that of V5 in the dorsal stream.

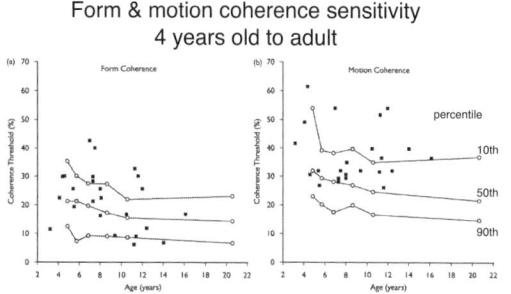

Gunn, Cory, Atkinson, Braddick, Wattam-Bell, Guzzetta, Cioni
NeuroReport 2002
Hemiplegics worse on motion then form
(black squares are individual hemiplegic children)

Direct comparison of form & motion coherence

both stimuli are made up of dots on circular arcs
they are presented in sequence for motion and simultaneously for form

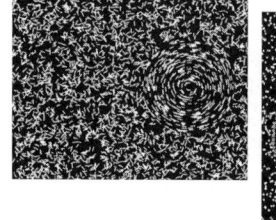
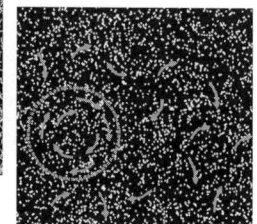

New 'ball in grass' (static or rotating) test

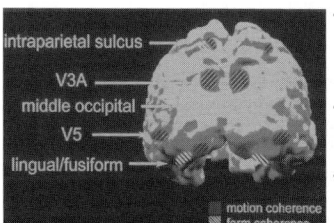

fMRI: coherent vs incoherent form & motion
Braddick et al (Current Biology, 2000)

- independent networks of areas responding to form coherence and motion coherence
- multiple areas outside V1 respond to global coherence in each case
- non-overlapping networks but not gross dorsal/ventral anatomical divide

form & motion coherence thresholds
- school groups + adults ball in the grass task

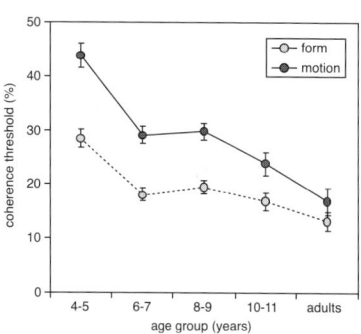

Form and motion coherence norms
concentric patterns

Figure 4.
Top left: Plot of coherence thresholds from behavioural measures, for form and motion for normally developing children and hemiplegic children against chronological age. The lines show the 10th, 50th and 90th percentiles for normal children. Individual hemiplegic children are the black squares.
Bottom left: fMRI schematic on normal adults for the form and motion coherence stimuli. Contrast is between coherent and incoherent.
Top right: schematic diagram of "ball in the grass" test with comparable stimuli, used in VEP studies on infants and for psychophysical studies on children, for measuring form and motion coherence.
Bottom right: normative data on "ball in the grass" test for normal children between 4 and 12 years and normal adults. Mean threshold measures.

We have previously identified from fMRI studies of normal adults, specific areas involved in our form and motion coherence tasks (Braddick et al., 2000; Braddick et al., 2001). A schematic of this result is shown in Figure 4. This work has shown that anatomically distinct circuits are activated in global processing of form and motion, although each circuit involve parts of both the parietal and temporal lobes, and cannot therefore be said to be strictly "dorsal" and "ventral" in the human brain. However, the activated areas do include dorsal stream areas V5 and V3A for motion, and anatomically ventral areas for form. It has also been found that the BOLD response in fMRI studies increases linearly with degree of coherence in an area analogous to V5 (Rees et al., 2000) and we find that areas in the lingual/fusiform gyrus, which may include V4, similarly show a linear response with form coherence (Braddick et al., 2002b).

The global form stimulus can be used in a preferential-looking method with infants, where the partially coherent circular configuration appears on one side of the display and a random array of line segments on the other. This method has demonstrated that 4-6 month olds show a significant but weak response to global form, which is absent in 2-month olds (Braddick et al., 2002a). Thus, although local orientation sensitivity emerges earlier in development than directional selectivity (Braddick, 1993; Atkinson et al., 2002d), global organization based on orientation is less effective in determining infant behaviour than global organization based on motion. This may reflect the importance of global motion for segmentation and depth organization of the visual world. Such segmentation arises both from the independent movement of objects, and from parallax due to self-motion; the latter is effective for infants even though their self-motion is largely passive rather than actively controlled in the first six months (Von Hofsten et al., 1992).

Global motion and dorsal stream vulnerability

As we have discussed above, signal/noise thresholds for coherent motion can be used as an index of dorsal stream function. In considering development and pathology, we need to identify delays or deficits that are specific to this system, as distinct from general attentional or other factors which may affect performance on a wide range of tasks. In a number of populations, therefore, we have compared motion coherence thresholds with the form coherence thresholds.

The first group we studied were young children (up to 15 years) with Williams Syndrome. This developmental disorder, related to a specific deletion on chromosome 7, shows a very characteristic cognitive profile, with relatively strong expressive language abilities combined with unusual semantic knowledge and social sensitivity, but very poor spatial cognition (see for example Braddick & Atkinson 1995; Bellugi et al., 1988; Bellugi et al., 1999; Klein & Mervis 1999; Atkinson et al., 2001). Within the visual domain children with Williams syndrome show relatively good ability to recognise faces (e.g. Bellugi et al., 1990) but marked sensory, visuomotor and visuocognitive deficits (e.g. see Braddick & Atkinson 1995; Atkinson et al., 2001). This profile suggests the possibility of a deficit in dorsal compared to ventral stream function. This is supported by our findings that, in a "mail-box" task comparing the ability to match perceptually the orientation of a slot with the control of an action posting a "letter" through the slot (Milner & Goodale, 1995), children with Williams syndrome show disproportionately poor performance on the latter, presumed dorsal-stream, function (Atkinson et al., 1997a). Many children with Williams syndrome in the same study showed a relative deficit in global motion *versus* form coherence thresholds. We have subsequently studied larger groups, both of children with Williams syndrome and typically developing controls (Atkinson et al., 2003c; Gunn et al., 2002) and find considerable variability in the group with Williams syndrome. While all children in the group showed that they understood the task, some showed performance in the normal range for their mental age, while others showed much poorer performance in the motion coherence than the form coherence task. Individuals with very high motion thresholds are also found in our group of normal 4-5 year olds. It is unlikely that the WS results represent a simple delay in development, since children who show this performance are scattered through the age range up to 15 years. Children with WS typically show very slow development of spatial tasks beyond the normal 3-6 year old level (*e.g.* Bellugi et al., 1999; Braddick & Atkinson, 1995; Atkinson et al., 2003b) and this may also be the case for the coherence tasks.

To evaluate the developmental end point of global motion sensitivity in Williams syndrome, it is useful to look at a group of affected adults. In comparison to normal adult controls, the adults with Williams syndrome showed a significantly greater deficit of performance on the motion coherence than on the form coherence test (Atkinson et al., 2003c).

However, deficits specific to global motion processing are not unique to Williams syndrome. Another clinical group we have studied with the same tests consisted of hemiplegic children with IQ performance in the normal range (see results in *Figure 4*). Despite their normal cognitive level, these children showed significantly poorer global motion performance for age than typically developing children, while their global form sensitivity was unaffected. (Gunn et al., 2002) A similar impairment of motion relative to form sensitivity has also been found in a group of autistic children (Spencer et al., 2000; O'Brien et al., 2002) and a motion coherence deficit has been found in studies of developmental dyslexia (Cornelissen et al., 1995; Ridder et al., 2001, Stein et al., 2000) and in children with fragile X (Kogan et al., 2004).

As this motion coherence deficit appears to be a common feature across a wide variety of paediatric disorders with very different aetiologies and neurodevelopmental profiles, we suggest that it represents an early vulnerability in the motion processing stream of a very basic nature. In the case of dyslexia, this has been described as the "magnocellular hypothesis" (Stein et al., 2000) although the relationship between the magnocellular system, as defined at the geniculate level, and the motion processing areas of the cortex is not straightforward. Closer comparison between behavioural, electrophysiological, and structural imaging data on brain development, in both normally developing children and those with developmental disorders, will be necessary to elucidate the brain modules and mechanisms underlying this "dorsal stream vulnerability".

■ Conclusion: Current neurobiological model of dorsal and ventral stream development

Figure 1 summarizes our main findings so far on the relative development of form processing and motion processing mechanisms, which can be thought of as functions of the ventral and dorsal cortical streams respectively.

We have reviewed evidence that the dorsal stream is more vulnerable in development. This comes from children aged 4 years and over, in whom the parsing of the visual array into globally organized forms appears to develop more securely than the equivalent parsing by relative motion. However, the course of these functions in early infancy appears to be more complex. Sensitivity to pattern properties (*e.g.* orientation) is apparent earlier in cortical development than to directional motion, perhaps because the latter is constrained by the need for precise temporal organisation of the inputs to visual cortex (Braddick *et al.*, 2005). No such constraint, however, prevents newborn control of OKN by a subcortical route.

The early orientation sensitivity we have described could reflect pattern processing at a quite local level, of the kind known to occur in V1. One aspect of more global processing that is present early is the sensitivity to face-like configurations (Johnson & Morton 1991; Simion *et al.*, 1998). However, it has been argued that this represents an initial subcortical process which biases the input to promote development of cortical selectivity (Johnson & Morton 1991). In contrast, infants' sensitivity to the segmentation of the field by oriented texture (Atkinson & Braddick 1993) is present at 12 weeks but not clearly before. Infants' preference for a globally defined concentric form over the same local elements randomly distributed is present, but weak, at 16 weeks and undetectable at 8 weeks (Braddick *et al.*, 2002a).

Thus orientation processing is present early but does not apparently lead to very salient global segmentation in infants. Motion sensitivity, in contrast, emerges later but segmentation by motion is sufficiently salient that it can be used in preferential looking to test individual infants' coherence thresholds (Wattam-Bell, 1994; Mason *et al.*, 2003). This may reflect the importance of differential motion in eliciting attention and fixation to an object in extra-foveal vision, compared to form processing as a function of central vision which may therefore be reflected better in other measures than preferential looking. Global motion processing has an important functional role in early life, but even so depends on a relatively delicate, vulnerable system whose disruption is apparent in a range of developmental disorders.

Of course, for effective visuo-cognitive and visuo-motor function, motion and form processing cannot operate in isolation from each other. Object motion must be perceptually bound to the identity of a recognized object, and motion yields information about 3-D shape and biological characteristics which may make essential contributions to object recognition. The binding of motion to object identity has been the subject of much discussion in relation to the development of object permanence. Hopefully, studies of development in the future will be able to provide a neurobiologically based account of how dorsal- and ventral-stream information are integrated, and perhaps more sensitive tools for understanding developmental anomalies.

ABCDEFV (Atkinson Battery of Child Development for Examining Functional Vision)

We have developed a test battery, solely for measurements of functional vision, for both children with normal and abnormal general development. We have devised the battery using ideas from paediatric neurology, ophthalmology, visual neuroscience and developmental psychology. We have included in the tests a number of recently developed new methods, adapted from research on visual development in infants and young children e.g. preferential looking, videorefraction. The battery spans the mental age range from birth to six years. Of course the chronological age of children completing the tests may be much wider than this age range, when clinical populations are involved.

The rationale of these tests is that different parts of the battery tap different aspects of sensory, perceptual, motor and cognitive vision. The battery is transportable, so that it can be used in different settings. We intend this battery as a diagnostic starting

Core vision tests

Test	Function assessed
1. Pupil responses	Responsiveness of pupils to light assessed as a basic indicator of neurological integrity.
2. Diffuse light reaction	Orientation to light as an indicator of minimal visual function in very young infants and cases of suspected total blindness.
3. Lateral tracking	Visual attention and eye movements (either saccadic or smooth pursuit accepted).
4. Peripheral refixation – lateral fields	Visual attention and extent of lateral visual fields.
5. Symmetrical corneal reflexes	Binocular alignment. Manifest strabismus may be associated with ocular and/or neurological problems.
6. Convergence to approaching object	Binocular function; failure may indicate neurological or ophthalmic problems.
7. Attention at distance	Sustained visual attention possible at moderate distance; failure may be related to distance acuity or to neurological attentional problems.
8. Defensive blink to approaching object	Development of visuo-motor response related to distance perception.
9. Visually follows falling toy	Visual cognition: early stage in development of object permanence.

Core vision tests (optional)

10. Optokinetic nystagmus	Reflex eye movements associated with subcortical mechanisms.
11. Acuity Cards	Measurement of visual acuity.
12. Videorefraction	Accommodation, attentional shifts and refractive error.

point for pinpointing areas of concern in visual development in individual children. Failure on particular tests will not necessarily address the total extent of the problem, but rather raise a marker, so that the child can be referred to the appropriate specialist. The tests are divided into core vision tests and additional tests, the idea being that all children complete the core vision tests and only a subset of the children will complete the additional tests because they are generally for children capable of reaching and grasping with both hands and of a perceptual and cognitive age of beyond 6 months (see table below for the individual tests). The tests and normalization have been fully described in several publications (*e.g.* Atkinson *et al.*, 1989*b*; Atkinson, 2000; Atkinson *et al.*, 2002*b*).

Additional tests

Test	Min age	Function assessed
13. Lang test	2 yr	Stereoscopic vision.
14. Batting/reaching	4 mo	Visuomotor development.
15. Pick up black and white cotton	12 mo	Visual control of fine hand and finger movement (including pincer grasp); crude test of contrast sensitivity.
16. Retrieval of partially covered object	6 mo	Visual cognition: intermediate stage in development of object permanence.
17. Retrieval of totally covered object	10-12 mo	Visual cognition: intermediate stage in development of object permanence.
18. Shape matching with form board	2 yrs	Shape recognition, recognition of spatial relations, visual planning and control of manual actions.
19. Embedded figures	2 yrs	Figure-ground segmentation and shape recognition.
20. Placing letter in envelope	2 yrs	Recognition of spatial relations, visual planning control of manual actions.
21. Block construction – free play	12 mo	Requires recognition of spatial relations, visual planning and control of manual actions.
22. Copying block designs	18 mo	Graded test of recognition of spatial relations, visual planning and control of manual actions. Identifies developmental problems of "constructional apraxia".

ABCDEFV – application in paediatrics

The tests are very suitable for children with West Syndrome, particularly around the time of diagnosis and over the first years of life, provided the child is motorically capable of reaching and grasping at least with one hand. We have used the ABCDEFV in various clinical groups:

Normal children with marked refractive errors

We have used the ABCDEFV to follow up normally developing children with marked refractive errors including hyperopia (long sight-spherical errors and astigmatism) at 9 months of age in a vision screening programme in Cambridge Health District. Here in the second programme we screened a population of around 5,000 healthy infants, representing 80% of infants born in the Distinct over a 2 year period (Anker et al., 2003). Around 5% of these children show significant hyperopia and were followed up at 6 monthly intervals to 7 years of age alongside a control group of normally developing infants without refractive errors recruited from the same Well Baby Clinics. We found that children who had been significantly hyperopic in infancy performed significantly worse than controls on a number of the visuoperceptual, visuo-cognitive and spatial tests in the ABCDEFV at 14 months and 3.5 years, although there were no significant overall differences between the groups on the Griffiths Child Development Scales, MacArthur Communicative Development Inventory and British Picture Vocabulary Scales (Atkinson et al., 2002a) where both groups performed in the normal range. Excluding those infants who became amblyopic and strabismic did not substantially alter these results, suggesting that the differences between groups were not a direct causal consequence of these early visual disorders, but that the failures had an underlying common cause across visual, visuomotor, visuocognitive and visuspatial domain. These results indicate that early hyperopia is associated with a range of developmental deficits that persist at least to age 5.5 years. These effects are concentrated in visuocognitive and visuomotor domain rather than the linguistic domain and may reflect consequences of early degraded visual input, and/or a mild neurological deficit that affects both refractive development, preschool vision and preschool development across these domains.

Children born prematurely before 32 weeks

We have also used the ABCDEFV to follow longitudinally a cohort of children born very prematurely (before 32 weeks gestation), referred for assessment from the neonatal unit in the Hammersmith Hospital. The behavioural results on ABCDEFV were compared with neonatal MRI analysis, in which the extent of white matter changes was categorized along a scale from mild/normal neonatal MRI to severe abnormal MRI in terms of DEHSI (see brief discussion above). This is "diffuse excessive high signal intensity" on T2 weighted images which is present in approximately 75% of images taken at term equivalent age in infants born less than 30 weeks gestation (Maalouf et al., 1999) and has been taken as a possible sign of abnormal myelination. Figure 4 shows both the comparison of imaging category with the core and additional tests from the ABCDEFV. There is a good correlation between the imaging data and category of abnormality from DEHSI. We find that many of the children with only mild indications of brain abnormality fail on the spatial tests of copying constructions of block designs and other visuocognitive tests, *e.g.* where the child has to identify embedded figures or match shapes in a puzzle (Atkinson 2002; Atkinson 2003; Atkinson et al., 2003a).

Tests of Frontal Lobe function-executive control of attention

Use of these tests with normally developing children, children with Williams syndrome and children born very prematurely

Counterpointing-inhibition of a prepotent response

The test of "antisaccades", in which participants are required to make a saccade in the opposite direction to a target, has been widely used to investigate higher levels of cortical control of eye movements in adult pathologies; in particular it is argued that problems with this task result from deficits in frontal mechanisms required to inhibit the prepotent fixation response (e.g. Pierrot-Deseilligny et al., 1989). However, this antisaccade task is difficult to explain and to monitor with young children. To test the ability to override a prepotent spatial orienting response, we have devised an analogous manual "pointing/counterpointing" task using the same stimulus display as in the fixation shifts paradigm, in which the child has to point to the target as it appears, or to the opposite side to where it appears (see *Figure 5*).

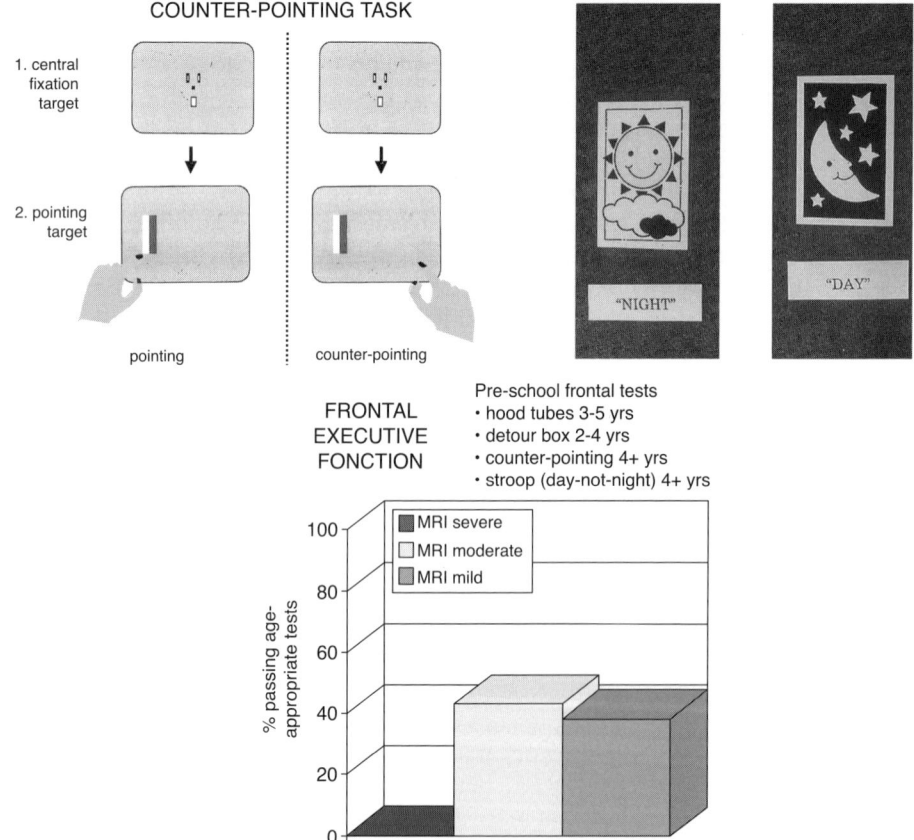

Figure 5.
Top left: schematic diagram of frontal test "counter-pointing" where the child has to point to the opposite side of the screen to where the stimulus black and white bar appears *i.e.* inhibit a pointing action...
Top left: schematic diagram of the cards used in frontal "Day-Night" Stroop test, where the child has to say the opposite word associated with the picture *i.e.* inhibit a verbal association.
Middle: three categories of premature infants according to severity of damage seen on neonatal MRI plotted against ability on frontal lobe executive control tests.

On each trial the child initially fixates a central face-like figure which alternates between 2 formats at 3 Hz. When the child is fixating, a target appears 13.5 cm either left or right of centre. The target consists of adjacent bright and dark stripes, each 2.9 cm wide by 14.7 cm high, reversing in contrast at 3 Hz. In 50% of trials ("competition" condition) the central figure remains visible; in the other 50% ("non-competition" condition) it disappears at the time of target onset. The pointing/counterpointing test is appropriate for children of a developmental age who can understand instructions to point towards and away from the targets (4 years and older mental age). In the pointing condition, the task is to point to the target as quickly as possible after it appears. Most young children find it easier to put their hand on the target, thus making the point explicit. In the counterpointing condition, when the target appears the requirement is to point as quickly as possible to the opposite side of the screen from the target. In either case, an observer watches the participant's actions on video and presses a button by which the computer records the latency to touch the screen. The pointing condition is tested first, starting with a demonstration and test that the child understands the task, followed by 20 trials. The counterpointing task is then introduced, if necessary with an explanation that "the computer is trying to catch you out – don't let it trick you, point to the other side from the stripes to make the stripes disappear". When the child has shown that they can perform this task, by giving three consecutive correct responses, 20 trials are run in the counterpointing condition.

We have used this test for measuring frontal lobe function in a large group of children with Williams syndrome (Atkinson et al., 2003b). In general they show marked delays on this inhibition task. In general their performance is well below their verbal mental age and in line with many other visuomotor and spatial skills. Many of these children never learn to consistently inhibit the prepotent responses of pointing to the target.

Detour Box and Day/night Frontal lobe tests of inhibition and attention

Detour box

This apparatus, originally devised by Hughes and Russell (1993) as a test of executive function in young and autistic children, consists of a box with an aperture at the front through which the child can see a brightly coloured ball on a platform. The tester explains to the child that this is a "magic box", and demonstrates that, if he or she reaches through the aperture to pick up the ball, the ball falls through a trapdoor in the platform and disappears from view. (This is achieved by the hand interrupting an invisible photocell beam which controls an electrically operated latch.) The tester then demonstrates that the ball can be obtained by a less direct method. In the lever task, a lever, mounted on a shaft coming through the side of the box, rotates a visible paddle which pushes the ball off the platform; the ball rolls down a chute into a tray where the child can pick it out. In the switch task, the paddle is locked so that the lever method does not work, but a switch on the other side of the box can be operated to inactivate the photocell and allow the ball to be retrieved directly by reaching out with the hand. In this condition, the activation of the photocell is signalled to the child by red lights on either side of the aperture. Because there is no visible connection between operating the switch and physical access to the ball in the switch task, young children find it harder than the lever task; normative data (Drake et al., 1993; Biro & Russell 2001) indicate that it is typically mastered by 3.5 years compared to 2.5 years for the lever task in normally developing children.

The lever task is tested first. The child is allowed to reach directly and sees the effect of interrupting the beam; the tester then reaches directly and shows that he/she gets the same effect. The tester then demonstrates three times how the ball can be retrieved successfully by operating the lever. The child is then encouraged to retrieve the ball. Each trial is scored as a correct response or as an error (direct reach, or no response until prompted). After an error, a child is reminded of the correct method. Trials continue until three successive correct responses are made (to a maximum of 15 trials). Performance is measured by the number of errors before this criterion is reached.

The switch task is then tested by a similar procedure. In this case, attempting to operate the lever counts as an error. Almost half the children with Williams syndrome (15/36) did not attain the performance of normal 3.5 year olds on the detour box

"Day-night" task

This is a variant of the Stroop test, devised by Gerstadt et al., (1994) to examine frontal control processes in normal children aged 3.5-7 years. The task requires children to overcome a familiar verbal response, by saying "day" to a card with a cartoon picture of the moon in a starry dark sky, and saying "night" to a cartoon picture of the sun among clouds in a bright sky (see *Figure 5*). The results are compared with a control task in which the responses "day" and "night" are arbitrarily assigned to patterns with no pre-existing associations (one card showing a red-green checkerboard, and another with a wavy stripe across each diagonal of the card). The sun-moon test is run first, with the tester demonstrating the correct responses, and then giving the child two practice trials, one with each card. Practice continues until the child had produced a correct response to each card at least once. Sixteen trials with the sun/moon cards in random order are then given, without feedback.

The great majority of children with Williams syndrome who can do the control task perform at or above the 5 year old level on the day-night test. When the data are plotted in terms of the vocabulary age equivalent, most of the children with Williams syndrome perform around, or above their verbal age equivalent level.

Relation between frontal tasks

IN Williams syndrome we can say that there does appear to be a general "frontal factor", in the sense that detour box and day-night performance are markedly correlated, even when the association with vocabulary age indexed by the BPVS is taken out. In addition the correlation of counterpointing with detour box performance appears substantially higher than that with day-night performance. The detour box test shows the clearest relationship to BPVS age.

The comparison of these frontal tasks makes it clear that, as well as considerable variation between individuals which is not closely tied to their chronological age, the performance of children with Williams syndrome on "frontal" tasks is highly task-dependent. A number of them did not show sufficiently secure associative learning on the control task, (showing many errors), for the day-night results to be revealing. However, the remainder performed the task at a level that was broadly in line with their verbal ability as reflected in vocabulary. In contrast, performance on the detour box showed a considerably greater deficit relative to controls across the majority of the group.

Frontal tests on premature infants

We have tested the premature children (described above) and in *Figure 5* show their performance against the severity of abnormality in white matter shown on neonatal MRI. Many of the children in all three MRI groups show marked deficits on these tasks. These tests have proved to be sensitive indicators of attention and executive function deficits in the preschool years and are highly likely to be predictive of later attentional problems.

These frontal tests would be highly appropriate for later testing of many children with West Syndrome and may give an early indicator of mild yet important deficits...

Conclusions

Our general conclusions so far from using these tests are that:

- Many infants born at term, with indications of perinatal brain damage on neonatal MRI, shows remarkable recovery of function, even with extensive damage to classical visual occipital areas. However, some parts of the cortical and subcortical visual systems show markedly less developmental plasticity than others. Damage seen on MRI in basal ganglia is a marker for poor recovery and is found even when occipital cortex is intact.

- Infants with early hemispherectomy show (i) lack of the FS attentional response under competition on their "bad" side of space; (ii) evidence for subcortical control in early life of the visual optokinetic responses for both directions of movement (OKN for pattern movement to left and right). However, after 5 months of age the direction which would normally involve control from the damaged hemisphere becomes non-functional despite the intact subcortical system.

- From fMRI studies on normal adults and measures of sensitivity to form and motion coherence in infants and children, we have demonstrated functioning of the two independent extrastriate visual subsystems. These are the "ventral" stream for perceptual recognition of shape, form, objects and faces and "dorsal" stream for spatial relations, relative movement and planning actions. A range of developmental disorders, including hemiplegia, Williams Syndrome, and Autism, show greater impairment of motion coherence than form coherence when compared to the normal developmental course. We propose the hypothesis of "dorsal stream vulnerability"
the dorsal system shows relatively less plasticity and is more vulnerable in development than the ventral system. This may also be true in West syndrome.

- We already know that significant prematurity is associated with poor visual and cognitive outcome, with visual problems being due to either or both development in the eyes and brain. In a number of centres (*e.g.* Volpe, de Vries, Marlow, Eken,

Cioni, Atkinson, Guzzetta) visual, motor and cognitive deficits have been found in premature infants with periventricular leukomalacia (PVL) with the additional finding that PVL is followed by reduced cortical grey matter at term (Inder et al., 2005). Healthy very low birth weight premature infants, who are normal on ultrasound and neurological examination, show normal timing of onset of visual cortical function, as indicated by a significant OR VEP at the appropriate age. (Atkinson et al., 1990; Braddick et al., 1989; Atkinson et al., 1989a; Atkinson et al., 2002c). However, in very premature infants with abnormalities on ultrasound this cortical response is delayed or absent (Atkinson et al., 2002c).

– In two large scale studies in progress, in collaboration with the neonatal teams at the Hammersmith Hospital, the OR-VEP and Fixation Shifts measures provide sensitive indicators for visual and general development and later neurological outcome. In addition, the ABCDEFV and tests of executive function in the frontal lobes, indicate marked visual and visuocognitive deficits associated with cystic PVL, with reduced incidence of abnormality in premature infants in the subgroups with abnormalities other than cystic PVL on MRI, and lesser problems again in the group with apparently relatively normal neonatal MRI (absence of moderate or severe DEHSI- diffuse excessive high signal intensity possibly related to lesser myelination).

– The preschool attentional tests (indicating developmental abnormalities within frontal and parietal lobes) provide very sensitive indicators for less severe problems and may be related to school age attentional disorders (ADHD). The FS test and other preschool attentional tests may prove valuable in gauging the effectiveness of early intervention for infants with potential perinatal brain damage, and children with developmental syndromes such as West Syndrome. These early measures may be useful in predicting later cognitive development and measuring the effectiveness of early intervention, whether it be pharmacological or educational.

In this chapter I have described a number of tests, both behavioural and electrophysiological which have been used successfully with clinical groups of varying disability from mild to severe. Many of them would be suitable for children in the early years with West syndrome to aid diagnosis at an early age, to measure the effects of intervention and drug treatment and to predict cognitive outcome at a later age.

Acknowledgements

Work described here was supported by Programme Grant G7908507 from the Medical Research Council. I thank my co-director, Professor Oliver Braddick, my co-principal investigator, Dr. John Wattam-Bell, and other colleagues both in and outside the Visual Development Unit, in particular Shirley Anker, Dr. Dee Birtles, Dr. Marko Nardini,(Visual Development Unit, UCL) Dr. Eugenio Mercuri, Professor Giovanni Cioni and Dr. Andrea Guzzetta whose work has contributed to these studies. In particular, I would like to thank Professor Franco Guzzetta for inviting me to contribute to this stimulating workshop on West Syndrome.

Visual Development Unit website http://www.psychol.ucl.ac.uk/vdu/publications/

References

Anker S, Atkinson J, Braddick O et al. Identification of infants with significant refractive error and strabismus in a population screening program using noncycloplegic videorefraction and orthoptic examiniation. *Invest Ophthalmol Vis Sci* 2003; 44: 497-504.

Atkinson, J. Human visual development over the first six months of life. A review and a hypothesis. *Human Neurobiol* 1984; 3: 61-74.

Atkinson, J. New tests of vision screening and assessment in infants and young children. In: French JH, Harel S, Casaer P, eds. *Child neurology and development disabilities*. Baltimore: Paul H. Brookes Publishing, 1989: 219-27.

Atkinson, J. Review of human visual development: Crowding and dyslexia. In: Cronly-Dillon J, series ed., Stein JF, vol. ed. *Vision and visual dysfunction: Vol. 13. Vision and visual dyslexia*. United Kingdom: MacMillan Press, 1991: 44-57.

Atkinson, J. Earlsy visual development: differential functioning of parvocellular and magnocellular pathways. *Eye* 1992; 6: 129-35.

Atkinson, J. The Cambridge assessment and screening of vision in high-risk infants and young children. In: Anastasiow NJ & Harel S eds. *At-risk infants: Interventions, families, and research*. Baltimore: Paul H. Brookes Publishing, 1993a.

Atkinson, J. Vision in dyslexics: Letter recognition acuity, visual crowding, contrast sensitivity, accommodation, convergence and sight reading music. In: Wright SF & Groner R, eds. *Facets of dyslexia and its remediation. Studies in visual information processing*. Elsevier Science Publishers B.V, 1993b: 125-38.

Atkinson, J. The "where and what" or "who and how" of visual development: An update of current neurobiological models. In: Simion F & Butterworth G, eds. *The development of sensory, motor and cognitive capacities in early infancy. From perception to cognition*. Hove, England: Psychology Press, 1998: 3-24.

Atkinson, J. *The developing visual brain*. Oxford: OUP (Oxford Psychology Series 32), 2000.

Atkinson, J. Visual consequences of periventricular leucomalacia. Paper presented at the XVIIth Neuroradiologicum Symposium, Paris, France, 2002.

Atkinson, J. Visual problems in premature infants. *Rev Neurol* 2003; 36: 569.

Atkinson J & Braddick OJ. Early development of the control of visual attention. *Perception* 1985; 14: A25.

Atkinson J, Braddick OJ. Visual segmentation of oriented textures by infants. *Behav Brain Res* 1993; 49: 123-31.

Atkinson J & Braddick O. Neurobiological models of normal and abnormal visual development. In: De Haan M, Johnson M, eds. *The cognitive neuroscience of development*. Hove, England: Psychology Press, 2003: 43-71.

Atkinson J & Braddick O. Dorsal stream vulnerability and autistic disorders: The importance of comparative studies of form and motion coherence in typically developing children and children with developmental disorders (Commentary on E. Milne, J. Swettenham, R. Campbell, "Motion perception and autistic spectrum disorder: A review"). *Cahiers de psychologie cognitive* (Current Psychology of Cognition) 2005; 23 (1-2): 49-58.

Atkinson J & Hood B. Deficits of selective visual attention in children with focal lesions. *Infant Behav & Dev* 1994; 17: 423.

Atkinson J & Hood B. Development of visual attention. In: Burack JA & Enns JT, eds. *Attention, development, and psychopathology*. Guildford Press, 1997: 31-54.

Atkinson, J & Mercuri E. Visual development in infants with neonatal focal brain lesions *Strabismus* 1995; 3: 178.

Atkinson J & Van Hof-van-Duin J. Visual assessment during the first years of life. In: Fielder A & M. Bax M, eds. *Management of visual impairment in childhood*. London: MacKeith Press, 1993.

Atkinson J, Anker S, Braddick O, Nokes L, Mason A & Braddick F. Visual and visuo-spatial development in young Williams Syndrome children. *Dev Med & Child Neurology* 2001; 43: 330-7.

Atkinson J, Anker S, Braddick O, Rutherford M, Edwards D, Cowan F. Deficits in selective visual attention and dorsal stream function: Children with hyperopic refractive errors in infancy and children born prematurely. *Invest Ophthalmol Vis Sci* 2004; 45: E-Abstract 3511.

Atkinson J, Anker S, Nardini M, et al. Infant vision screening predicts failures on motor and cognitive tests up to school age. *Strabismus* 2002a; 10: 187-98.

Atkinson J, Anker S, Rae S, Hughes C, Braddick O. A test battery of child development for examining functional vision (ABCDEFV). *Strabismus* 2002b; 10: 245-69.

Atkinson J, Anker S, Rae S, Weeks F, Braddick O, Rennie J. Cortical visual evoked potentials in very low birthweight premature infants. *Arch Dis Child Fetal Neonatal Ed* 2002c; 86: F28-F31.

Atkinson J, Braddick OJ, Anker S, et al. Visual development in the VLBW infant. In: *Transactions of the IVth European Conference on Developmental Psychology*, University of Stirling, 1990: 193.

Atkinson J, Braddick OJ, Anker S, et al. Visual development in the VLBW infant. In: *Transactions of the 3rd Meeting of the Child Vision Research Society*. Rotterdam, 1991.

Atkinson J, Braddick O, Anker S, et al. Early visual marker tasks indicating abnormal visual development in very premature infants. *Invest Ophthalmol Vis Sci* 2003a: 44

Atkinson J, Braddick O, Anker S, et al. Extending the "dorsal stream vulnerability hypothesis": Spatial reorientation and motion and form coherence in children and adults with Williams syndrome. *J Vision* 2003; 3: Abstract 287a.

Atkinson J, Braddick O, Anker S et al. Extending the "dorsal stream vulnerability hypothesis": Spatial reorientation and motion and form coherence in children and adults with Williams syndrome. *J Vision* 2003; 3: Abstract 287a.

Atkinson J, Braddick OJ, Wattam-Bell J. Infant cortical mechanisms controlling OKN, saccadic shifts, and motion processing. *Invest Ophthalmol Vis Sci* 1993; 34: 1357.

Atkinson J, Braddick OJ, Wattam-Bell J, Hood B, Weeks F. Temporal-frequency and orientation selectivity of orientation-specific responses in young infants. *Perception* 1989a; 18: 492.

Atkinson J, Gardner N, Tricklebank J, Anker S. Atkinson Battery of Child Development for examining functional vision (ABCDEFV). *Ophthalm Physiol Optics* 1989b; 9: 470.

Atkinson J, Hood, B, Braddick OJ, & Wattam-Bell J. Infants' control of fixation shifts with single and competing targets: Mechanisms of shifting attention. *Perception* 1988; 17: 367-8.

Atkinson J, Hood B, Wattam-Bell J & Braddick OJ. Changes in infants' ability to switch visual attention in the first three months of life. *Perception* 1992; 21: 643-53.

Atkinson J, King J, Braddick O, Nokes L, Anker S, Braddick F. A specific deficit of dorsal stream function in Williams Syndrome. *NeuroReport* 1997a; 8: 1919-22.

Atkinson J, King J, Braddick OJ, Nokes L, Anker SE & Braddick F. Dorsal visual stream dysfunction in Williams' Syndrome: Deficits in motion coherence and visual control of action. *Invest Ophthalmol Vis Sci* 1997b; 38: S223.

Atkinson J, Mercuri, E, Braddick, et al. Development of orientation processing and visual attention in infants with perinatal cortical and/or basal ganglia damage on MRI. *Invest Ophthalmol Vis Sci* 1998; 39: S884.

Atkinson J, Macpherson F, Rae S, Hughes C. Block constructions in young children: Development of spatial grouping ability. *Strabismus* 1994a; 2: 41.

Atkinson J, Wattam-Bell J, Braddick O. Development of directional and orientational-selective VEP responses: Relative functional onset of dorsal and ventral stream processing in human infants. *Invest Ophthalmol Vis Sci* 2002d; 43: E-Abstract 3992.

Atkinson, J, Weeks F, Anker, S, Rae, S, Macpherson F, Hughes, C. VEP and behavioural measures for delayed visual development in VLBW infants. *Strabismus* 1994b; 2: 42.

Banton T, Bertenthal BI, Seaks J. Infants' sensitivity to statistical distributions of motion direction and speed. *Vision Res* 1999; 39: 3417-30.

Baranello G, Rando T, Bancale A et al. Auditory attention at the onset of West syndrome: Correlation with EEG patterns and visual function. *Brain Dev* 2006; 28: 293-9.

Bellugi U, Sabo H, Vaid J. Spatial deficits in children with Williams syndrome. In: Stiles-Davis J, Kritchevsky M, Bellugi U, eds. *Spatial Cognition: Brain bases and development.* Hillsdale NJ: Lawrence Erlbaum, 1988: 273-98.

Bellugi U, Bihrle A, Trauner D, Jernigan T, Doherty S. Neuropsychological, neurological, and neuroanatomical profile of Williams syndrome children. *Am J Med Genet* (suppl), 1990; 6: 115-25.

Bellugi U, Lichtenberger L, Mills D, Galaburda A, Korenberg JR. Bridging cognition, the brain, and molecular genetics: Evidence from Williams syndrome. *Trends Neurosci* 1999; 22: 197-207.

Biagioni E, Cioni G, Cowan F et al. Visual functions and EEG reactivity in infants with perinatal brain lesions at 1 year. *Dev Med Child Neurol* 2002; 44: 171-6.

Biro S, Russell J. The execution of arbitrary procedures by children with autism. *Dev Psychopathol* 2001; 13: 97-110.

Braddick OJ. Orientation- and motion-selective mechanisms in infants. In: Simons K., ed. *Early visual development: Normal and Abnormal. Committee on Vision, Commission on Behavioral and Social Sciences and Education, National Research Council.* New York: Oxford University Press, 1993.

Braddick OJ, Atkinson J. Visual and visuo-spatial development in young Williams Syndrome children. *Invest Ophthalmol Vis Sci* 1995; 36 (suppl): S954.

Braddick O, Qian N. The organisation of global motion and transparency. In: Zanker JM & Zeil J, eds. *Motion vision.* Berlin: Springer Verlag, 2000: 86-112.

Braddick O, Atkinson J, Hood B, Harkness W, Jackson G, Vargha-Khadem F. Possible blindsight in infants lacking one cerebral hemisphere. *Nature* 1992; 360: 461-3.

Braddick OJ, Atkinson J, Julesz, B, Kropfl W, Bodis-Wollner I, Raab E. Cortical binocularity in infants. *Nature* 1980; 288: 363-5.

Braddick OJ, Atkinson J, Wattam-Bell, J. Development of visual cortical selectivity: binocularity, orientation, and direction of motion. In: von Euler ed. *Neurobiology of early infant behaviour.* London: MacMillan, 1989: 165-72.

Braddick O, Atkinson J, Wattam-Bell J. Normal and anomalous development of visual motion processing: Motion coherence and "dorsal stream vulnerability". *Neuropsychologia* 2003; 41: 1769-84.

Braddick O, Birtles D, Wattam-Bell J, Atkinson J. Motion- and orientation-specific cortical responses in infancy. *Vision Res* 2005; 45: 3169-79.

Braddick O, Curran W, Atkinson J, Wattam-Bell J, Gunn A. Infants' sensitivity to global form coherence. *Invest Ophthalmol Vis Sci* 2002e: 43: E-Abstract 3995.

Braddick OJ, O'Brien J, Rees G, Wattam-Bell J, Atkinson J, Turner R. Quantitative neural responses to form coherence in human extrastriate cortex. Paper presented at the annual meeting of the Society for Neuroscience (Program no. 721.9), 2002.

Braddick OJ, O'Brien JMD, Wattam-Bell J, Atkinson J, Turner R. Form and motion coherence activate independent, but not dorsal/ventral segregated, networks in the human brain. *Curr Biol* 2000; 10: 731-4.

Braddick OJ, O'Brien JMD, Wattam-Bell J, Atkinson J, Hartley T, Turner R. Brain areas sensitive to coherent visual motion. *Perception* 2001: 30: 61-72.

Braddick OJ, Wattam-Bell J, Atkinson J. Orientation-specific cortical responses develop in early infancy. *Nature* 1986; 320(6063): 617-9.

Braddick, OJ, Wattam-Bell J, Day J, Atkinson J. The onset of binocular function in human infants. *Hum Neurobiol* 1983; 2: 65-9.

Cornelissen P, Richardson A, Mason A, Fowler S, Stein, J. Contrast sensitivity and coherent motion detection measured at photopic luminance levels in dyslexics and controls. *Vision Res* 1995; 35: 1483-94.

Damasio, AR, Benton AL. Impairment of hand movements under visual guidance. *Neurology*, 1979; 29: 170-8.

de Haan, M, Johnson MH, Halit H. Development of face-sensitive event-related potentials during infancy: A review. *Intl J Psychophysiol* 2003; 51: 45-58.

de Haan M, Pascalis O, Johnson MH. Specialization of neural mechanisms underlying face recognition in human infants. *J Cogn Neurosci* 2002; 15; 14 (2): 199-209.

Drake J, Lee S, Russell J. *The development of detour-reaching ability in toddlers*. Undergraduate dissertation, Department of Experimental Psychology, Cambridge University, 1993.

Gallant JL, Braun J, Van Essen DC. Selectivity for polar, hyperbolic, and Cartesian gratings in maxaque visual cortex. *Science* 1993; 259: 100-3.

Gerstadt CL, Hong YJ, Diamond A. The relationship between cognition and action: Performance of children $3\,{}^1/_2$-7 years old on a Stroop-like day-night test. *Cognition* 1994; 53: 129-53.

Gunn, A, Cory E, Atkinson J, et al. Dorsal and ventral stream sensitivity in normal development and hemiplegia. *Neuroreport* 2002; 13 (6): 843-7.

Guzzetta F, Frisone MF, Ricci D, Rando T, Guzzetta A. Development of visual attention in West syndrome. *Epilepsia* 2002; 43: 757-63.

Hood B, Atkinson J, Braddick OJ, Wattam-Bell J. Visual attention shifts in infants and neurologically impaired children. *Ophthal Physiol Opt* 1989; 9: 472.

Hood B, Atkinson J. Dissociating sensory visual loss from cognitive deficits in the selective attention system of normal and neurologically impaired infants. *Transactions of the IVth European Conference on Developmental Psychology*, University of Stirling, 1990: 184.

Hood B, Atkinson J. Sensory visual loss and cognitive deficits in the selective attentional system of normal infants and neurologically impaired children. *Dev Med Child Neurol* 1990; 32: 1067-77.

Hughes C, Russell J. Autistic children's difficulty with mental disengagement from an object: Its implications for theories of autism. *Dev Psychol* 1993; 29: 498-510.

Inder, TE. Warfield SK, Wang H, Huppi PS & Volpe JJ, Abnormal cerebral structure is present at term in premature infants. *Pediatrics* 2005; 115 (2): 286-194.

Johnson MH, Morton J. *Biology and Cognitive Development: The Case of Face Recognition*. Oxford: Blackwell, 1991.

Klein BP, Mervis CB. Contrasting patterns of cognitive abilities of 9 and 10 year-olds with Williams syndrome or Down syndrome. *Dev Neuropsychol* 1999; 16: 177-96.

King J. Dissociation of ventral and dorsal visual processing in Williams Syndrome. Paper presented at the meeting of the Experimental Psychology Society, Cardiff, UK, 1997.

Kogan CS, Bertone A, Cornish K et al. Integrative cortical dysfunction and pervasive motor perception deficit in fragile X syndrome. *Neurology* 2004; 63: 1634-9.

Livingstone M, Hubel DH. Segregation of form, color, movement and depth: anatomy, physiology and perception. *Science* 1988; 240: 740-9.

Maalouf EF, Duggan PJ, Rutherford MA et al. Magnetic resonance imaging in a cohort of extremely premature infants. *J Pediatr*. 1999; 135: 351-7.

Mason AJS, Braddick O, Wattam-Bell J. Motion coherence thresholds in infants – different tasks identify at least two distinct motion systems. *Vision Res* 2003; 43(10): 1149-57.

Maunsell JHR, Newsome WT. Visual processing in monkey extrastriate cortex. *Ann Rev Neurosci* 1987; 10: 363-401.

Maunsell JH, Van Essen DC. Topographic organization of the middle temporal visual area in the macaque monkey: Representational biases and the relationship to callosal connections and myeloarchitectonic boundaries. *J Comp Neurol* 1987: 266: 535-55.

Maunsell JHR, Van Essen DC. Functional properties of neurons in middle temporal visual area of the macaque monkey I. Selectivity for stimulus directions, speed and orientation. *J Neurophysiol* 1983; 49: 1127-47.

Maunsell JHR, Van Essen DC. Functional properties of neurons in middle temporal visual area of the macaque monkey II. Binocular interactions and sensitivity to binocular disparity. *J Neurophysiol* 1983; 49: 1127-47.

Mercuri E, Anker S, Guzzetta A et al. Neonatal cerebral infarction and visual function at school age. *Arch Dis Child Fetal Neonatal Ed* 2003; 88: F487-91.

Mercuri E, Anker S, Guzzetta A et al. Visual function at school age in children with neonatal encephalopathy and low Apgar scores. *Arch Dis Child Fetal Neonatal Ed* 2004; 89: F258-62.

Mercuri E, Atkinson J, Braddick O, et al. Visual maturation in children with focal brain lesions on neonatal imaging. *Neuropediatrics* 1995; 26: 348.

Mercuri E, Atkinson J, Braddick O, et al. Visual function and perinatal focal cerebral infarction. *Arch Dis Childhood* 1996; 75: F76-F81.

Mercuri E, Atkinson J, Braddick O et al. Visual function in full-term infants with hypoxic-ischaemic encephalopathy. *Neuropediatrics* 1997; 28: 155-61.

Mercuri E, Atkinson J, Braddick O et al. Basal ganglia damage in the newborn infant as a predictor of impaired visual function. *Arch Dis Childhood* 1997; 77: F111-F114.

Mercuri E, Atkinson J, Braddick O et al. Chiari I malformation and white matter changes in asymptomatic young children with Williams Syndrome: Clinical and MRI study. *Eur J Paed Neurol* 1997; 5/6: 177-81.

Mercuri E, Atkinson J, Rutherford M et al. Maturation of visual function in infants with HIE. *Transactions of the British Paediatric Neurology Association XXII Annual Meeting.* Southampton, 1996.

Mercuri E, Braddick O, Atkinson J et al. Orientation-reversal and phase-reversal visual evoked potentials in full-term infants with brain lesions: A longitudinal study. *Neuropaediatrics* 1998; 29: 1-6.

Mercuri E, Haataja L, Guzzetta A et al. Visual function in full term infants with brain lesions: correlation with neurologic and developmental status at two years of age. *Brain Dev* 1998; 20: 336.

Mercuri E, Haataja L, Guzzetta A et al. Visual function in term infants with hypoxic-ischaemic insults: Correlation with neurodevelopment at 2 years of age. *Arch Dis Child Fetal Neonatal Ed* 1999; 80: F99-F10

Milner AD, Goodale MA. *The visual brain in action.* Oxford, England: OUP, 1995.

Morrone MC, Atkinson J, Cioni G, Braddick OJ, Fiorentini A. Developmental changes in optokinetic mechanisms in the absence of unilateral cortical control. *NeuroReport* 1999; 10: 1-7.

Morton J, Johnson MH. CONSPEC and CONLERN: A two-process theory of infant face recognition. *Psychol Rev* 1991; 98: 164-81.

Newsome WT, Paré EB. A selective impairment of motion processing following lesions of the middle temporal area (MT). *J Neurosci* 1988; 8: 2201-11.

O'Brien J, Spencer J, Atkinson J, Braddick O, Wattam-Bell J. Form and motion coherence processing in dyspraxia: Evidence of a global spatial processing deficit. *Neuroreport* 2002; 13: 1399-402.

Pierrot-Deseilligny C, Rivaud S, Gaymard B, Agid Y. Cortical control of reflexive visually-guided saccades. *Brain* 1989; 114: 1473-85.

Rando T, Bancale A, Baranello G et al. Visual function in infants with West syndrome: correlation with EEG patterns. *Epilepsia* 2004; 45: 781-6.

Rando T, Baranello G, Ricci D et al. Cognitive competence at the onset of West syndrome: correlation with EEG patterns and visual function. *Dev Med Child Neurol* 2005; 47: 760-5.

Ridder WH, Borsting E, Banton T. All developmental dyslexic subtypes display an elevated motion coherence threshold. *Optomet Vis Sci* 2001; 78: 510-7.

Spencer J, O'Brien J, Riggs K, Braddick O, Atkinson J, Wattam-Bell J. Motion processing in autism: Evidence for a dorsal stream deficiency. *NeuroReport* 2000; 11: 2765-7.

Stein J, Talcott J, Walsh VV. Controversy about the visual magnocellular deficit in developmental dyslexics. *Trends Cogn Sci.* 2000; 4: 209-11.

Turati C, Simion F, Milani I & Umilta C. Newborns' preference for faces: What is crucial? *Dev Psychol* 2002; 38 (6): 875-82.

Ungerleider LG, Mishkin M. Two cortical visual systems. In D. J. Ingle, MA Goodale, RJW Mansfield (eds.) *Analysis of Visual Behavior*, Cambridge, MA: MIT Press, 1982: 549-86.

Von Hofsten C, Kellman P, Putaansuu J. Young infants sensitivity to motion parallax. *Infant Beh & Dev* 1992; 15: 245-64.

Wattam-Bell J. Analysis of infant visual evoked potentials (VEPs) by a phase-sensitive statistic. *Perception* 1985; 14: A33.

Wattam-Bell J. Coherence thresholds for discrimination of motion direction in infants. *Vision Research* 1994; 34 (7): 877-83.

Wattam-Bell J. Displacement limits for the discrimination of motion direction in infancy. *Invest Ophthalmol Vis Sci* 1991; 32 (suppl) (4): 964.

Zeki SM. Functional organization of a visual area in the posterior bank of the superior temporal sulcus of the rhesus monkey. *J Physiol* 1974; 236: 549-73.

Zeki S. Functional specialization in the visual cortex of the rhesus monkey. *Nature* 1978; 274: 423-8.

Zeki S. The distribution of wavelength and orientation selective cells in different areas of monkey visual cortex. *Procs Roy Soc B* 1983; 217: 449-70.

Zeki S. Color coding in the cerebral cortex – the reaction of cells in monkey visual cortex to wavelengths and colors. *Neuroscience*, 1983; 9: 741-65.

Zeki S. *A Vision of the Brain*. Oxford: Blackwell Scientific, 1993.

Zihl J, von Cramon, D & Mai N. Selective disturbance of motion vision after bilateral brain damage. *Brain* 1983; 106: 313-40.

Developmental features in West syndrome

Thierry Deonna, Hélène Chappuis, Danièle Gubser-Mercati, Anne-Lise Ziegler, Eliane Roulet-Perez

Unité de Neurologie et de Neuro-réhabilitation pédiatrique, Département médico-chirurgical de Pédiatrie, CHUV, Lausanne, Suisse

---

West syndrome is considered the prototype of "epileptic encephalopathy" a term implying that the epileptic activity itself (and not only the underlying brain disorder or antiepileptic therapy) contributes to an acquired cerebral pathology (an encephalopathy) with behavioral and developmental consequences, both during the active epileptic period, but often also permanently after epilepsy has remitted.

The marked behavioral effects of the unique type of cerebral dysrhythmia observed on the EEG (diffuse, with continuous multifocal disorganized electric activity known as hypsarrhytmia) and their improvement when therapy suppresses this have been well recognized since the first clearly effective treatment (ACTH) was found in the early 1960's (Sorel, 1958). This could not be observed before that period, and the developmental prognosis was thought to be almost uniformly poor (Illingworth, 1955; Jeavons, 1970).

In a minority of babies who had been developmentally normal until the onset of epilepsy and in whom no cause could be found (the so-called "idiopathic cases", 15-30% of all cases) one can observe the potentially devastating effect of the epileptic disorder (Illingworth, 1955). This is even more striking in those slightly older babies in whom sometimes enough normal development has been present before the epilepsy started. In such cases, one can see the dramatic change in alertness, interpersonal contact, and emotional reactivity with stagnation in developmental progresses or even a regression followed by progressive recovery, coinciding with the remission of spasms and normalization of the EEG.

More recently, one has realized that some babies with definite brain lesions, such as prenatal or perinatal cerebral infarcts or even with malformations (*i.e.* some cases of tuberous sclerosis) who develop typical West syndrome can have a good, sometimes even normal cognitive development after the epilepsy is controlled despite a history of regression and possible long stagnation after the onset of the disease (Alvarez, 1987; Golomb, 2005). These cases indicate that the ultimate prognosis does not depend only on the consequences of the pre-existing brain pathology or that of the epilepsy "alone". An important implication here is that whatever underlying brain pathology there might be (and we now know that there is often one, even if not shown by the most modern technics), and provided the baby was normal or almost normal prior to the onset of epilepsy, development can resume if the epileptic disease is controlled (or occasionally has stopped spontaneously).

The duration of the epileptic activity and its age at onset prior to diagnosis and therapy is considered a crucial factor for prognosis. This factor has however been difficult to appreciate for two main reasons. First is the fact that many subtle, progressive and fluctuating behavioral signs of the epileptic activity can occur (disturbed sleep, decreased social interactions, irritability) before the spasms are recognized (Kellaway,1979). Secondly, once epilepsy has started, it may be of variable duration and severity, with periods of spontaneous remission and recurrence during several months. Comparisons between babies with early and late diagnosed West syndrome show a better outcome for those with early diagnosis, effective therapy and short duration of spasms (Kivity, 2004). Such comparisons can only be done in babies with reasonably good early development (the cryptogenic cases), because the effect of the epileptic variable is difficult to appreciate in those with severe brain disease and pre-existing retardation. Due to the small number of cases for such comparisons, it has understandably been difficult to demonstrate statistically and unequivocally the major effect of early and long-standing West syndrome which is observed clinically.

An important old observation repeatedly made by experienced clinicians is that some of the babies who had a stagnation or regression but were successfully treated (or occasionally whose epilepsy remitted spontaneously) have a prolonged period of slow development in the following months or even years before they progress at a faster pace and recover to a normal or fairly good level. This dynamics of development is rarely documented but is remarkable, and there have been few neuropsychological and developmental studies of such situations. This lack of data is to be contrasted with the several number of studies on long term cognitive outcome now available. These have confirmed the predictive value of certain clinical factors (normal development prior to onset of spasms, rapid control of spasms, absence of demonstrable brain disease) which had already been recognized since ACTH became a routine treatment in the early 1960s (Sorel, 1958).

To better understand the influence of this early form of epilepsy on development and behavior in the acute stage and how "recovery" takes place during the following first months or years after disease control both in terms of its time course and of its impact on different developmental fields, two conditions must be present. First, it is necessary to observe these children longitudinally as early as possible and with frequent controls and prolonged follow-ups. Secondly, they should not be too severely affected developmentally before disease onset so that a measurable progress can be expected and measured in the early months and later following cessation of the epileptic symptomatology. Such studies are rarely possible, although they might shed light on questions regarding the effects on the developing brain of the seizures and the bioelectrical dysfunction on the EEG:

1) Is there really a long time-lag after epilepsy has remitted before developmental "catch-up" is seen and 2) Can one demonstrate clearly that it occurs and until when a full normalization is possible? 3) During the recovery period, can one show different cognitive-behavioral patterns of dysfunctions reflecting selective involvement of localized cortical regions affected by the epileptic disorder or preferential vulnerabilities of some systems (attentional for example)?

Better knowledge of these questions is both theoretically and practically relevant. First, it helps to understand what this type of epilepsy does to developing brain systems and to what extent the consequences of this unique epileptic pathology can be compensated for in the best circumstances.

On the practical side, when evaluating the benefits and side-effects of antiepileptic therapy in this syndrome, it is of paramount importance to take into account these developmental issues.

In this chapter, we are reporting longitudinal observations made over several years in some babies with West syndrome, in each of whom a unique set of circumstances allowed to approach some of the above questions.

■ Personal studies

Cognitive follow-up of 12 children with West syndrome and normal development prior to onset of epilepsy (ALZ)

In 1991, one of us (ALZ) retrospectively analysed in great detail the clinical records of 12 babies born between 1971 and 1988 who had been diagnosed and treated at the CHUV for West syndrome, and whose development had been considered normal by history prior to the diagnosis. This included 11 babies with no specific neurological diagnosis or neurological signs and one with tuberous sclerosis, but who was developmentally normal. We wondered if the duration of epilepsy prior to diagnosis and treatment made a difference in developmental prognosis and seizure outcome. In trying to separate the cases according to the time elapsed from first spasms to diagnosis-therapy, we found 10 babies who had had spasms for less then 4 months and 2 for more then 10 months. Of the latter two, one was retarded and the other severely autistic. The other 10 children had an IQ or DQ above 80 at an age between 2 years and 14 years. Five of the 12 children have remained seizure-free and 5 later had partial epilepsy (2 of the retarded-autistic children, the one with tuberous sclerosis but, interestingly, two with normal development who in later childhood presented with resistant temporal lobe epilepsy, one with cortical dysplasia at epilepsy surgery).

This personal experience taught us several things. First it confirmed, what was at the time only beginning to be appreciated, that the existence of a demonstrable pathology was not equivalent to an ominous mental prognosis but that the quality of development prior to the epileptic disease was a good prognostic factor, providing the epilepsy could be controlled. We also found how difficult it was to know by history the real time onset of this epilepsy, because apathy, developmental stagnation, irritability, poor sleep were sometimes the initial, and fluctuating signs of the epileptic disease long before the spasms were recognized. This explains why it is almost impossible, given the small number of cryptogenic cases in a population of babies with infantile spasms to prove statistically that early diagnosis and therapy are a determining factor in prognosis.

This is true despite the fact that the marked deterioration in behavior and subsequent recovery with seizure control and suppression of the epileptic EEG activity makes it clinically so evident.

Longitudinal follow-up of two babies with cryptogenic West from age 5-6 months to age 2 ½ years (*Figures 1a* and *1b* and comments of methods)

Case MG: This 8 months old baby was seen with a history of typical spasms for since about a month.

The parents and paediatrician considered that the development had been normal and that there was no clear stagnation, but when we saw him at 8 months, the developmental level was at about 5-6 months. EEG showed typical hypsarrythmia. MRI was normal. Vigabatrin(VGB) 100 mg/kg was given and spasms subsided in 48 hours and did not recur. The control EEG 2 weeks later showed disappearance of the hypsarrhythmic pattern. The parents noted a clear improvement in alertness within a week. He was regularly followed in the outpatient clinic at 8 months, 11 months, 14 months, 20 and 30 months and a full developmental assessment was made with the parents using the Denver Developmental Screening Test (DDST, Frankenburg, 1967) each time. Repeated EEGs at 14 and 20 months were normal and VGB was gradually decreased after 7 months of remission and completely stopped at 19 months of age without recurrence of seizures up to the present age (3 years).

Case L.P. This boy was diagnosed at 6 ½ months with typical infantile spasms of one month duration and during this period "smiled less and less" with no clear regression preceding the diagnosis.

Development had been normal previously and cerebral MRI was normal. EEG showed typical hypsarrhythmia. VGB 75 mg/kg was given with marked decrease of spasms and total disappearance when increased to 100 mg/day. Control EEG after 3 weeks of therapy showed disappearance of hypsarrhythmia. VGB was gradually decreased

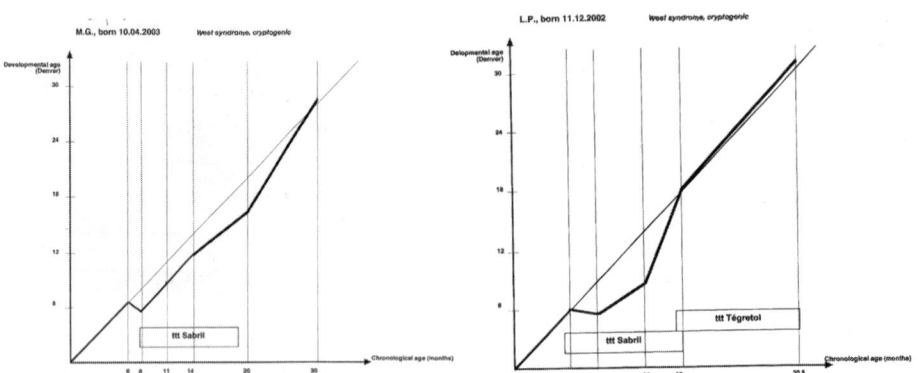

Figure 1. Longitudinal early developmental follow-up of two babies with cryptogenic infantile spasms. 1a: case MG. 1b: case LP.

from the age of 11 months and stopped at 18 months when carbamazepine was introduced. Repeated EEGs at 10 months, 14 months and 18 months showed no recurrence of hypsarrhythmia, but occasional spikes in the left frontotemporal area at 18 months.

He was followed in the outpatient clinic at 8 months, 14 months, 18 months and 30 months with the DDST.

■ Method of developmental study

At each visit, the Denver developmental screening test was administered by the paediatrician under the supervision of the author (TD) in the presence of both parents and in case LP with the help of the special education teacher who followed the child at home regularly. In the DSST, for each developmental item of the four domains tested (behavior-personal-social, fine motor-adaptation, language, and gross motor) there is an age range at which 25%, 50%, 75% and 90% respectively of normal children are able to succeed it. Each performance is either witnessed or enquired from the parents. Information on most of the items could be filled up unequivocally. For each item, the age at which 50% of children are able to perform was taken as the average developmental age, which was calculated at each age the child was seen and plotted against chronological age.

■ Results

Figure 1a shows the developmental pattern from the diagnosis of epilepsy. In case 1, as soon as epilepsy was controlled, development resumed, but remained below average for age (50th percentile) until about $2 \, ^1/_2$ years. According to the parents also, he made increasingly more rapid progress in each successive 3 to 6 months period. In case 2, although he had made definite progress between each visit, *Figure 1b* shows that he lagged below average (50th percentile) until 18 months of age. The speed of progress was clearly increased in the last 6 months compared to the equivalent time period. This confirmed the parents' impression that he had made more rapid progress in the last period.

Comment

These two cases are typical examples of cryptogenic infantile spasms with good therapeutic response. They clearly show a time delay between cessation of hypsarrhythmia and recovery with an initial slow pace of progress and acceleration later on. Our clinical impression and the result of the DSST did not show a significant heterogeneity between the different developmental fields.

Different impact of partial epilepsy *vs* epileptic spasms on behavior and devclopment? A case of tuberous sclerosis *(Figure 2)*

Case report: A.T. was diagnosed at 3 months with complex partial seizures (fixed gaze, automatisms and hypotonia) with the physical stigmata and typical MRI findings of tuberous sclerosis. Her behavior and development were absolutely normal for that

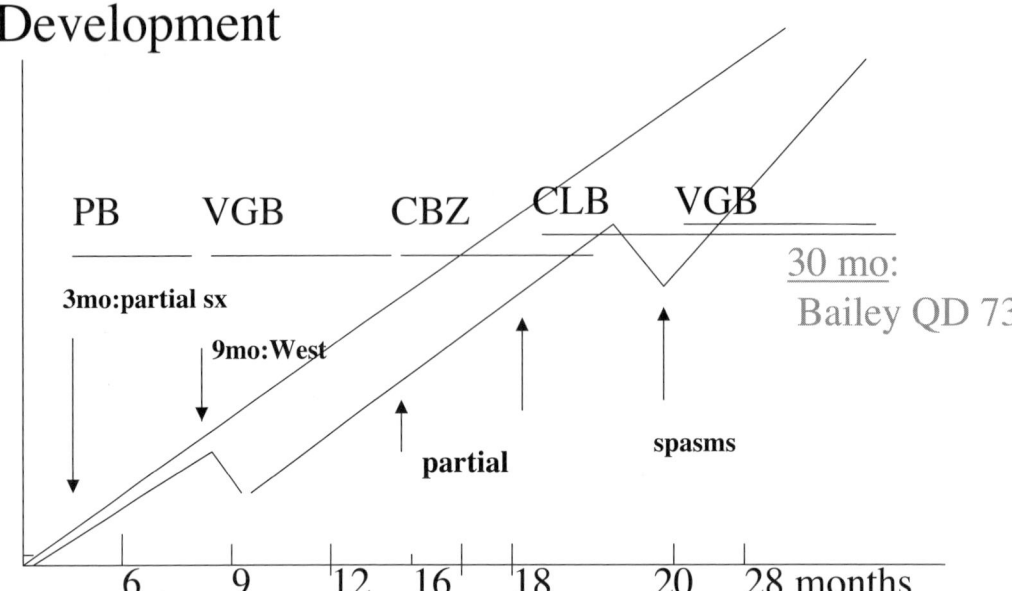

Figure 2. Case AT. Tuberous sclerosis with partial seizures and later two periods with hypsarhythmia. Clinical course. (See text).

age and the EEG showed only a right frontal spike focus. She was put on Phenobarbital with no recurrences and she continued to have normal development until 9 months of age when she developed typical spasms and hypsarrhythmia on the EEG. This had been preceded by a decrease in social interaction in the previous two weeks. VGB was given with full clinical and EEG response and the behavior was normal again. At 18 months of age, VGB was switched to carbamazepine, influenced in this decision by the initial good response of the partial seizure with Phenobarbital and to minimize the period on VGB treatment. At 20 months, she regressed again with recurrence of spasms and hypsarrythmia. After a brief period of clobazam, VGB was re-instituted with again a good response and she was maintained on monotherapy with this drug.

Since then she only has rare partial seizures and has continued to progress quite well, considering the basic diagnosis and early seizure onset, with a DQ of 73 on the Bailey Scale at the age of 2 ½ years.

Comment

Infantile spasms can occur in association with other types of seizures, mainly partial seizures, either at different periods in the evolution of the epileptic disorder, or at the same period (Gaily, 1995, Donat, 1991). When these occur together, it is difficult to separate the possibly different behavioral and developmental effects of the two seizure types in the same infant. In this case of tuberous sclerosis, we could observe her development (normal) while she had only simple partial seizures from the age of 3 to 9 months and how the change to epileptic spasms and hypsarrythmia on the EEG at 9 and 20 months (rapidly suppresssed with VGB) manifested at each period with a change of behavior and developmental stagnation. We could see the clearly negative effects of the epileptic spasms while the early partial seizures had not interfered significantly with her behavior. Of course this may vary according to the site of cortical onset and mode of spread of the partial seizures.

Case Y.P: Late infantile spasms: Longitudinal study (18 months to 3 ½ years) after delayed diagnosis, severe regression with marked stereotypies and significant late recovery after successful therapy (*Figure 3* and *Table I*)

Y.P. This girl, the second child of healthy parents, was referred to us at the age of 18 months with a diagnosis of epilepsy and severe developmental delay. Axial spasms with falls were observed and the EEG showed hypsarrhythmia. She exhibited incessant purposeless motor activity (walked alone at 14 months), no active object prehension, no imitation, a primitive social contact with smiles and gaze shifts towards people and going to her mother to be held, no play or language.

She had severe multiple hand stereotypies with hands in hands, hand to mouth, tapping surfaces, scratching, "polishing", reminiscent of Rett syndrome. Physical examination, statural and head growth were normal. Other abnormal behaviors included biting, hair pulling, pica, and running constantly without purpose. On the early Social and Communication Scale (ESCS), her level was at the 2 months. On the Bailey scale at 21 months, she had a Developmental Quotient of 27.

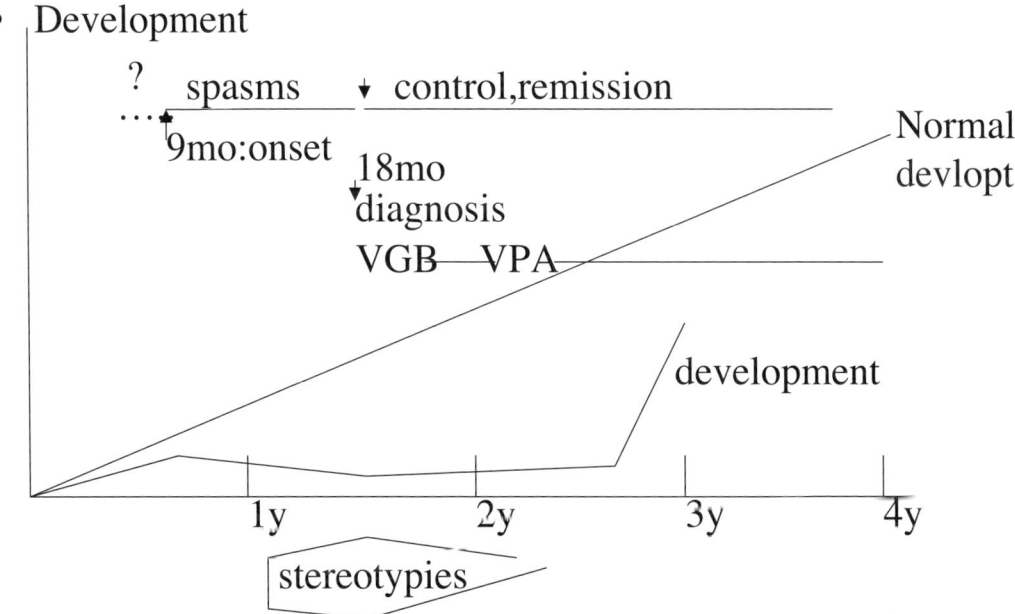

Figure 3. Y.P.: Summary of general evolution of the disorder showing delayed diagnosis, time of diagnosis, long stagnation, DQ obtained and course of stereotypies. For details see results.

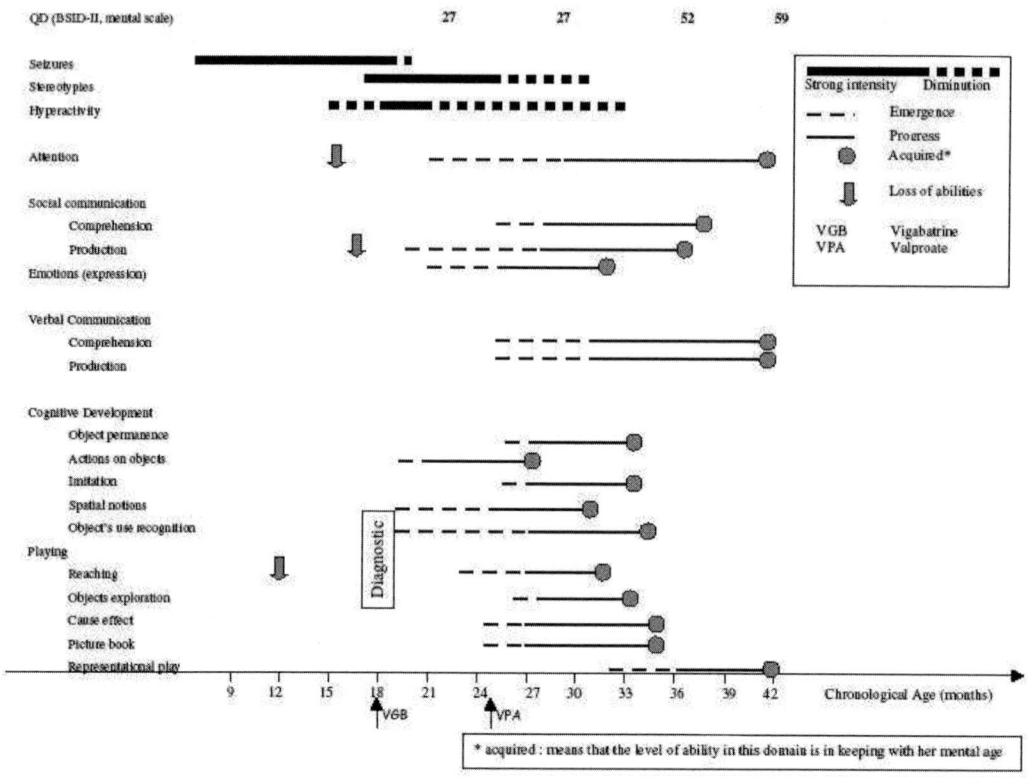

Table I. P.Y.: Time scale of developmental events before and after the diagnosis of epilepsy

Before 18 months, data are only historical (with one family video), whereas from 18 months they are a combination of different more objective sources (see method and case report).

She was given Vigabatrin 100 mg/kg/day and spasms disappeared completely within days. Within one to two weeks, a marked decrease in purposeless motor agitation, a slight decrease in stereotypies and more time in visual contact were noted by the family.

After two weeks of treatment, she started to show direct voluntary prehension of objects. Control EEG showed total disappearance of the hypsarrhythmic pattern and rare focal spikes in posterior regions. VGB was continued for a total of 7 months and replaced by Valproate 300 mg per day which she has been taking since then. There have been no recurrence of seizures in the 2 $^{1}/_{2}$ years follow-up and no sleep problems. EEGs were repeated at 21 months, 22 months, 27 months, 35 months and 48 months each time with a sleep recording. There was never a relapse of hypsarrhytmia, no focal or diffuse slowing, nor a generalized spike or spike wave pattern. There were occasional rare focal spikes in some tracings but no electroclinical seizures. At the last recording there were isolated spikes in the left frontoprecentral region. The diagnostic work-up included MRI (normal) search for MECP-2 mutation and a metabolic screen (normal).

Method of developmental study from 18 months to 3 ½ years

Intensive enquiry was made to understand how and why this probably long standing history of seizures and severe delay had not been recognized and to reconstruct her developmental history.

Parents were repeatedly questioned and family videos were reviewed. Her motor development had been quite normal (walked alone at 14 months), but communication was delayed from early on, with no clear imitation, no play or language. Family videos at 14 months showed her looking and smiling at her grand-mother, going to her on all fours when stimulated to go in a given direction and going to parents to be cuddled. From 13 months on, she regressed with agitation, irritability, and development of increasingly frequent stereotypies. The earliest probable seizure occurred at 9 months and consisted in a series of "yawning" followed by isolated head drop and fatigue, initially thought of as a game or habit. From 12 months on, yawning was followed by a axial spasms and from the age 14 months clusters of axial spasms in series and of increasing frequency occurred, at this time not preceded by other behaviors.

We made the hypothesis that her marked retardation and autistic behavior might be mainly the result of a prolonged severe and persistent epileptic activity from at least 9 months of age and that some or even a significant developmental potential could emerge providing that the epilepsy came under control and that environmental stimulation and educative support was given. Two questions were raised. 1) Can development resume if epilepsy is controlled, what will be the dynamics of the changes and will one observe a dissociation between different developing abilities, even if only temporarily so, and within which time frame. 2) Are the stereotypies related to the epileptic activity or a behavioral sign accompanying her severe brain dysfunction. 3) Can one compare this situation to that of a child with severe congenital mental retardation who has a 5 ½ month developmental level at the age of 18 months? For these reasons, we decided to document as precisely and frequently as possible her evolution.

Regular telephones with the family, home visits (ALZ and HC), clinical controls with the referring neuropaediatrician (DGM) were made and a preestablished grid containing possible acquisitions to be expected was given to the special education teacher to fill in during her weekly home visits to the family. Questionnaires (Portage, ESCS, Belsky, Sauvage, Uzgiris-Hunt) were used and a standardized test (Bailey: BSID-II) was administered and videotaped at 22, 24, 37 months and 42 months. A combination of all available data was used to document the approximate age at which a new behavior or ability was first noticed and how long it took to progress until it was considered as being mastered.

Result

The first sign of clinical improvement was related to general behavior (decrease of purposelesss motor agitation, increased attention time) and to a gradual decrease and then total disappearance of the hand stereotypies. By history, their onset and progression correlated with the activity of the epilepsy and their progressive cessation followed its control (13 to 25 months). It was not directly linked to the EEG paroxysmal activity, that is they were not "epileptic stereotypies" or epileptic automatisms.

No significant cognitive recovery was observed in the next 6 to 9 months following cessation of seizures as shown by the results on the Bailey Developmental Quotient, mental scale (DQ) *(Figure 3)* with very low unchanged scores at 21 and 27 months (DQ 27). After that, surprisingly, rapid progresses were seen and a DQ of 52 was obtained at 37 months and 59 at 42 months.

Table I shows the age at first emergence, the progression in the domains of communication, emotions and basic cognitive processes from 18 months on, keeping in mind that at that age, she had no other abilities except walking and distinguishing perhaps living from non-living creatures and smiling indiscriminately. At 22 months, she showed pleasure, fear, and anger, but no signs of social comprehension or initiative to communicate. At that age, she had acquired some object recognition, spatial notions and means to obtain objects, so that there was developmental dissociation with relative delay in social and interpersonal communication. From the beginning of the 3rd year, she progressed rapidly in these latter domains.

Comment

Despite the catastrophic developmental status when first seen, a totally unexpected and significant improvement occurred after both clinical epilepsy and hypsarrhythmia were controlled. There was a prolonged stagnation (6 to 12 months) with onset of significant and increasingly rapid developmental progress thereafter. This long stagnation can not be explained by a persistent undiagnosed epileptic activity (for instance during sleep), because repeated EEG (with sleep recording) during this period did not show any, and none of the seizures that parents were familiar with were seen after antiepileptic therapy was started. At 22 months, one could see no signs of either verbal or non-verbal comprehension, no active initiative to communicate or search for physical contact, whereas she had acquired some basic recognition of objects, spatial notions and "action means", so one could have described her as a severely retarded child with autistic features. From the beginning of the 3rd year, she progressed rapidly in emotional and interpersonal communication so that she was not in the autistic spectrum anymore. We are aware that a new developmental milestone or behavior is often the result of co-emerging capacities which gradually unfold. It is thus difficult to decide the exact age at which the child has clearly mastered them *(Table I)*.

However, we believe that the recovery profile seen after a prolonged severe epileptic dysfunction in an immature brain (which at one point stops completely) is so rarely observable that the attempted description is warranted.

Spontaneous recovery or unrecognized spasms with marked initial delay. Longitudinal study from 13 months to 4 years (case R.E., *Figure 4* and *5*)

R.E. a 13 month girl was referred for developmental delay and suspected autism. On examination she had a developmental level below 6 months of age and had no active communication or emotional reactivity. Parents gave a history of episodes strongly suggestive of infantile spasms at the age of 3, 6 and 8 months with regression and improvement in between. A sleep and waking EEG done two days after the consultation was normal and the rest of the neurological work-up was non-diagnostic. Two months later, her communication had surprisingly very much improved. At this time, review of the videofilm made during the initial consultation at 13 months showed a typical axial myoclonic seizure which had been overlooked *(Figure)*. Follow-up showed a regular catch-up with a transient language delay and a performance IQ of 84 (WPPSI-R) at 4 years 8 months.

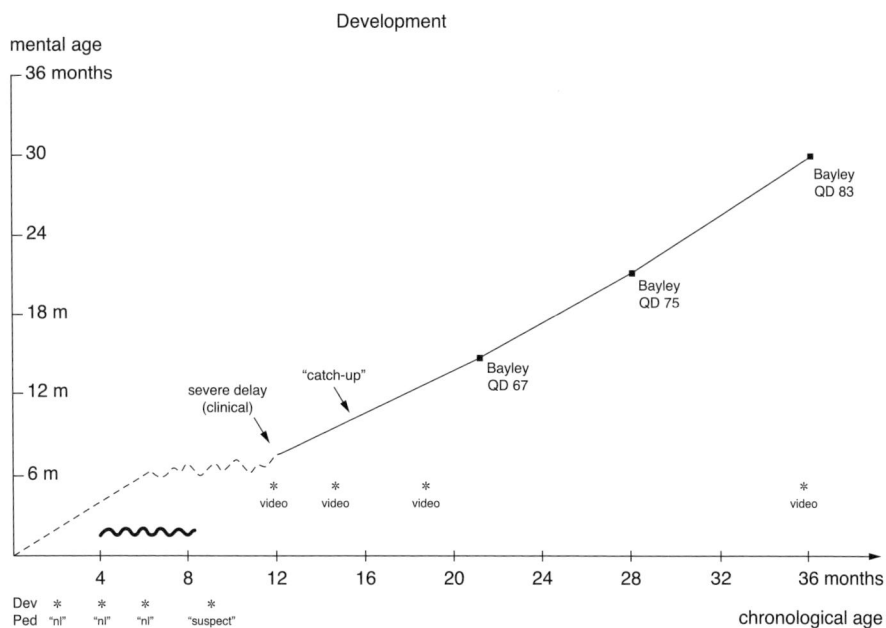

Dev.Ped : paediatrician's assessment with child considered normal("nl") , "suspect ": 9 months= first time when child's development considered suspect curved line: suspected spasms by history. *videos made.On the 1st one at 13 months an epileptic spasm was seen (se fig).

Figure 4. R.E: Clinical summary of case ER with developmental evaluation up to the age of 4 years (see case report).

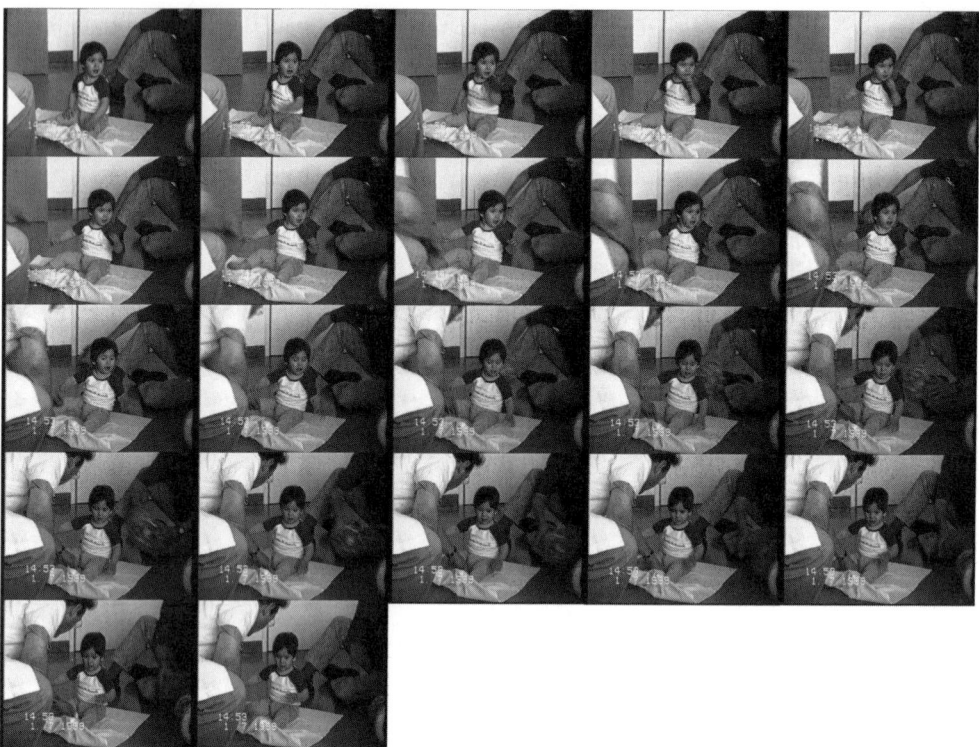

Figure 5. Case RE. Montage of a video-recorded axial spasm during the outpatient consultation.
The whole sequence of images lasts for 2 seconds. It starts with a brisk eye elevation (up row, 4th from left) and myoclonic jerk form the trunk with arm elevation, loss of balance and almost falling backward followed by recovery of normal posture and gaze.

Comment

The developmental "recovery" curve was remarkable in that the child came out of a state of severe delay (less than 6 months at 13 months) with an absence of communication and affective reactions with the surprising emergence in the next 3 months of basic communication behaviors (looking, giving, pointing) followed by progressive developmental acquisitions with improving DQ scores from 22 months to 36 months. At this age, she had an isolated language delay which normalized at the age of 4 years. At that age, the IQ on the WISC-R was 84. We are fully aware that in this case, the diagnosis of infantile spasms was purely clinical (documented spasm at 13 months on video and history of infantile spasms in infancy) and that the only EEG performed was normal. Such an outcome was totally unexpected and difficult to explain except as being due to temporary epilepsy (epileptic spasms) which could only be demonstrated clinically (the family refused a repeat EEG after the "spontaneous" recovery.

Discussion

The longitudinal observations we have presented suggest the following comments.

The developmental curves in the two babies who recovered from cryptogenic West syndrome indeed showed an initial slow phase before development accelerated significantly as one moved away from the acute epilepsy period. This, to our knowledge has not been fully documented before and should be further studied and confirmed. The lack of such data is however quite understandable for several reasons. Infant tests, their practical implementation and repeat administration carry their own logistic problems. One may also consider that this pattern of development has little significance considering the marked natural variability in normal babies. Behavioral side-effects of drugs (especially when ACTH was the only therapy) can mask developmental gains, another source of difficulty to discourage this type of study. In our cases, improvement started as soon as the children were given VGB and the developmental curve was not clearly influenced by its presence. Finally, the choice of the DSST and its value must be discussed. We are aware that the DSST is a screening and not a neuropsychological assessment tool. However, it consists of a lot of common, easily observable behaviors with well established norms of usual appearance in early years. When repeatedly performed using the same method to calculate an average (50th%) developmental age (see method), it gave us a reasonable idea of the developmental dynamics in our two children. With these limitations, we think that the trend seen in our two cases is noteworthy.

This trend was more clearly shown in the follow-up of the two other reported children (case Y.P and R.E.).

Can one explain the unique developmental course in YP and RE? It is possible that there was "freezing" of brain maturation that resumed after epilepsy stopped, or alternatively that there was a reorganization of ongoing developmental programs after epileptic damage. Of course it may be simply, but less likely, the effect of a slower recovery occurring in a previously abnormal brain.

However, a child with a diffuse congenital brain disease causing such a severe retardation at 18 months would not be expected to make such important progresses during that same time period. We also know that a transient delay can be seen after static early focal brain lesions. For instance, longitudinal studies done from the first months of life after congenital focal brain lesions have shown a transient delay in language development in the first years (from 1 to 3-4 years), which is later fully compensated for between 5 and – 6 years of age (Bates, 1992). One can therefore think that a combination of different factors may account for the unusual recovery patterns seen in the children we reported, some directly linked to the epilepsy ("Status epilepticus") during the active period, epileptic "damage" to developing networks; Huttenlocher, 1974) and others due to the basic underlying brain disorder and its inherent consequences, whose severity may be very different from one child to another.

A comment must be made on the severe stereotypies that followed the course of epilepsy in child P.Y. with onset, increase and resolution occurring in parallel with the control of epilepsy, but starting to disappear earlier than the period when developmental progresses became significant. Their resolution however did not occur abruptly and they persisted for some time after seizures were controlled. They can not be considered as direct epileptic manifestations or automatisms (videoEEG did not show a clear correlation either), but rather to the release of primitive patterns of movements due to the epileptic process. In fact the absence of voluntary prehension and the Rett-like hand stereotypies made us seriously consider this possibility initially. However, the search fot the mutation was negative and the evolution ruled out this diagnosis.

We wondered whether cases such as Y.P are extremely rare or simply not reported. Neville in 2001 published a Letter to the Editor (Neville, 2001) about a child with a remarkable long-term outcome after West syndrome diagnosed and treated at 8 months and marked developmental delay until late full recovery. At 3 years, the child "could not understand speech or recognize visually his mother". At 3.5 years, "speech appeared" and there was gradual recovery. At 4.5 years, the family thought that the "child had returned". At 12 years, psychological testing showed above average performances.

Neville interpreted the marked delay in the major developmental spheres as an epileptic auditory and visual agnosia. Long term follow-up studies of babies with West syndrome indicates that the outcome is not clear-cut between those who fully recover (normal) and those with permanent mental retardation. In fact, various specific learning or behavioural problems can be seen in children who are not retarded (high functioning autism, language disorders, etc.). Whether this is related to the basic causal brain pathology or to the direct effects of early epileptic "lesions" in some specific networks is difficult to know and both can probably occur (Asane, 2005).

Further behavioral and neuropsychological studies during the symptomatic acute period and during recovery are justified (Guzzetta, 1993, 2002, and chapter in this volume) to better document the developmental effects (global *versus* dissociated effects) of this particular epilepsy.

It should also be pointed out that epileptic spasms also occur (but much more rarely) beyond the first months of life (so-called late infantile spasms) during the second year of life. Some of these infants are already at a more advanced developmental stage, so that the role of epilepsy in the loss of functions is easier to see and document and because previously acquired skills can possibly recover better (Deonna and Roulet-Perez, 2005). Such situations offer a unique opportunity for developmental studies of these early epilepsies.

On the practical side, the implications of our observations for antiepileptic therapy should be discussed. While we now have two effective agents (ACTH-steroids and VGB), the question remains of their relative superiority in terms of time to cessation of spasms and EEG normalization and also in terms of side-effects, immediate and delayed. This has been looked for in a large multicentric study in Great Britain. A measure of comparison also used by these authors was the developmental outcome, first reported at 14 months (of course only in the idiopathic group) and very recently at 4 years of age in the babies treated with either ACTH-steroids or VGB (Lux, 2005; Darke, 2006). The variable dynamics of recovery suggested by our observations and the often specific deficits (and preserved domains) observed as the child grows up will need to be recognized when choosing time for final outcome measures and assessment tools as well as in the interpretation of results.

References

Asano E, Juhasz C, Shah A et al. Origin and propagation of epileptic spasms delineated on electroencephalography. *Epilepsia* 2005; 46: 1086-97.

Bates E, Thal D, Janowsky JJ. Early language development and its neural correlates. In: Segalowitz J.J. Rapin I. (Eds): *Handbook of neuropsychology*, vol 7, New York: Elsevier 1992: 69-110.

Bednarek N, Motte J, Soufflet C, Plouin P, Dulac O. Evidence for late infantile spasms.*Epilepsia* 1998; 39: 55.

Caraballo RH, Fejerman N, Bernardina BD, Ruggieri V, Medina C, Pociecha J. Epileptic spasms without hypsarrhythmia, *Epilept Disord* 2003: 109-13.

Chugani HT, Da Silva E, Chugani DC Infantile spasms: III. Prognostic implications of bitemporal hypometabolism on positron emission tomography. *Ann Neurol* 1996; 39: 643-9.

Deonna T, Roulet-Perez E. *Cognitive and behavioural disorders of epileptic origin in children*. Clinics in Developmental Medicine N° 168. Mac Keith Press Cambridge Univ. Press 2005.

Donat JF, Wright FS. Unusual variants of infantile spasms *J Child Neurol*, 1991; 6: 313-8.

Favata I, Leuzzi V, Curatolo P: Mental outcome in West syndrome. Progostic value of some clinical factors. *J Men Def Res* 1987; 31(Pt 1): 9-15.

Gaily E, Appelqvist K, Kantola-Sorsa E et al. Cognitive deficits afetr cryptogenic infantile spasms with benign seizure evolution. *Dev Med Child Neurol* 1999; 41: 660-4.

Gaily EK, Shewmon A, Chugani HT, Curran JG. Asymetric and asynchronous infantile spasms, *Epilepsia* 1995; 36: 873-82.

Glaze DG, Hrochovy RA, Frost JD Jr et al.: Prospective study of outcome of infants with infantile spasms treated during controlled studies of ACTH and prednisone. *J Pediatr* 1988, 112: 389-96.

Golomb MR, Carvalho KS, Garg BH. A 9 year-old with a history of large perinatal stroke, infantile and high academic achievement, *J Child Neurol* 2005; 20: 444-6.

Guzzetta F. Crisafulli A. Isaya Crine M. Cognitive assessment of infants with West syndrome. How useful in diagnosis and prognosis? *Dev Med Child Neurol* 1993, 35: 379-87.

Guzzetta F, Frisone MF, Ricci D, Randò T, Guzzetta A. Development of visual attention in West syndrome. *Epilepsia* 2002; 43: 757-63.

Huttenlocher PR. Dendritic development in neocortex of children with mental defect and infantile spasms. *Neurology*1974; 24: 203-10.

Illingworth R.S. Sudden mental deterioration with convulsions in infancy. *Arch Dis Child* 1955, 30: 529-37.

Jambaqué I, Mottron L, Chiron C. Neuropsychological outcome in children with West syndrome: a "human model" for autism. In: I. Jambaqué, M. Lassonde, O. Dulac. *Neuropsychology of childhood epilepsy* New York, Boston, Dordrecht, London, Moskow: Kluwer Academic/Plenum Publishers 2001; pp. 175-84.

Jeavons PM, Harper JR, Bower BD. Long term prognosis in infantile spasms: a follow-up report on 112 cases. *Dev Med Child Neurol* 1970; 12: 413-21.

Kellaway P, Hrachovy RA, Frost JD Jr, Zion T. Precise characterization and quantification of infantile spasms. *Ann Neurol* 1979; 6: 214-8.

Kivity S., Lerman P., Ariel R. Danziger Y, Mimouni M, Shinnar S. Long-term cogntive outcomes of a cohort of children with cryptogenic infantile spasms treated with high-dos Adrenocorticotropic hormone *Epilepsia*, 2004; 45: 255-62.

Koo B, Hwang PA, Logan WJ. Infantile spasms: outcome and prognostic factors of cryptogenic and symptomatic groups, *Neurology* 1993; 43: 2332-7.

Lombroso CT. A prospective study of infantile spasms:clinical and therapeutic correlations. *Epilepsia* 1983; 24: 135-58.

Lux AL, Edwards SW, Hancock E *et al.* The United Kingdom Infantile Spasms Study (UKISS) comparing hormone treatment with vigabatrin on developmental and epilepsy outcomes to age 14 months: a multicentre randomised trial. *Lancet Neurol* 2005; 4: 712-7.

Matsumoto A, Watanabe K, Negoro T, *et al.* Long-term prognosis after infantile spasms: A statistical study of prognostic factors in 200 cases. *Dev Med Child Neurol*, 1981; 23: 51-65.

Neville BG, Spratt HC, Birtwustle J. Early onset epileptic auditory and visual agnosia with spontaneous recovery associated with Tourette's syndrome. *J Neurol Neurosurg Psychiatry* 71: 560-1.

Riikonen R: A long-term follow-up study of 214 children with the syndrome of infantile spasms. *Neuropediatrics* 1982; 13: 14-23.

Riikonen R. Long-term outcome of patients with West syndrome. *Brain Dev*; 2001; 23: 683-7 Sorel L, Dusaucy_Bauloye A. A propos de cas d'hypsarrhythmie de Gibbs: son traitement spectaculaire par l'ACTH. *Acta Neurol Belg* 1958; 58: 130-41.

Sorel L, Dusauc Y, Bauloye A. À propos de cas d'hypoarrhythmie de Gibbs : son traitement spectaculaire par l'ACTH. *Acta Neurol Belg* 1958: 130-41.

West syndrome: epilepsy-induced neuro-sensory disorders and cognitive development

Franco Guzzetta

Child Neurology, Catholic University, Rome, Italy

Mental arrest or regression is one of the symptoms of the triad defining West syndrome (Commission on Paediatric Epilepsy of the ILAE, 1992). Nevertheless, studies on mental development in the acute stage of the disease are scanty and the symptom itself, as indispensable in West diagnosis at onset, is questioned (Lux and Osborne, 2004).

Poor mental outcome is more frequent among cryptogenic forms[1]. Characteristically, whatever the form, sensory changes of central origin (neurosensory signs) seem to herald the syndrome and their meaning has increasingly intrigued physicians and scientists.

■ Neurosensory impairment at the onset of spasms

At the onset of spasms a characteristic loss of eye contact, which is in most cases the first reason for medical referral, even more often than the perception of spasms itself, is observed. This abnormality of visual behaviour has been described decades ago by the first studies based on behavioural observation (Illingworth, 1955; Dongier *et al.*, 1964) and subsequently on neurophysiological techniques. Visual evoked potentials (VEP) were found to be transiently missing during the acute stage in a little cohort of West syndrome, as a sort of functional "blindness" (Wenzel, 1987). This impairment concerned especially the pattern-VEPs suggesting a rather specific cortical dysfunction. In particular, a mid-frequency depression of potentials evoked by sinusoidal alternating gratings of various spatial frequencies was observed in babies with infantile spasms, clearly showing a disorder of cortical visual function (Taddeucci *et al.*, 1984).

---

1. We will call cryptogenic all the cases without structural brain changes or signs of neurological disorder or a history of risk factors for neurological pathology, independently from the definition of probably idiopathic or probably symptomatic epilepsy.

A transitory cerebral visual impairment, recovering at least partially after the acute stage, has also been described in infants with West syndrome, suggesting a possible cortically mediated dysfunction (Castano et al., 2000). Similar patterns of visual regression in infantile spasms were also confirmed by other authors (Brooks et al., 2002).

Impaired neurovisual function has been described in cryptogenic West to be associated with perfusion defects in parieto-occipital regions using single photon emission computerized tomography (SPECT) (Jambaqué et al., 1993). The same parieto-occipital involvement was shown by Chugani et al. (1990) using positron emission tomography (PET) in some patients with the initial diagnosis of cryptogenic West; they were successfully treated with lobar resections whose neuropathological examination showed focal dysplasia (Chugani et al., 1993).

The association of visual abnormalities with EEG occipital slow waves and epileptiform discharges has been indicated as possible predictor of West syndrome in brain-injured infants before the appearance of spasms and hypsarrhythmia (Iiinuma et al., 1994; Suzuki et al., 2003). In some cases visual and cognitive deterioration has been observed some weeks before the onset of spasms, possibly representing a subtle early manifestation of epileptic encephalopathy (Jambaqué, 1993; Guzzetta et al., 2002). Accordingly, it has been suggested that the parieto-occipital regions may represent age-dependent sensitive areas involved in the mechanism of infantile spasms, especially when their onset is very early (Koo and Hwang, 1996) *(Figure 1)*.

Cortical visual function was recently studied in West syndrome using the fixation shift test (Guzzetta et al., 2002). This test aims at examining the cortical visual skill of shifting the gaze towards a novel visual stimulus, either in free scanning or in

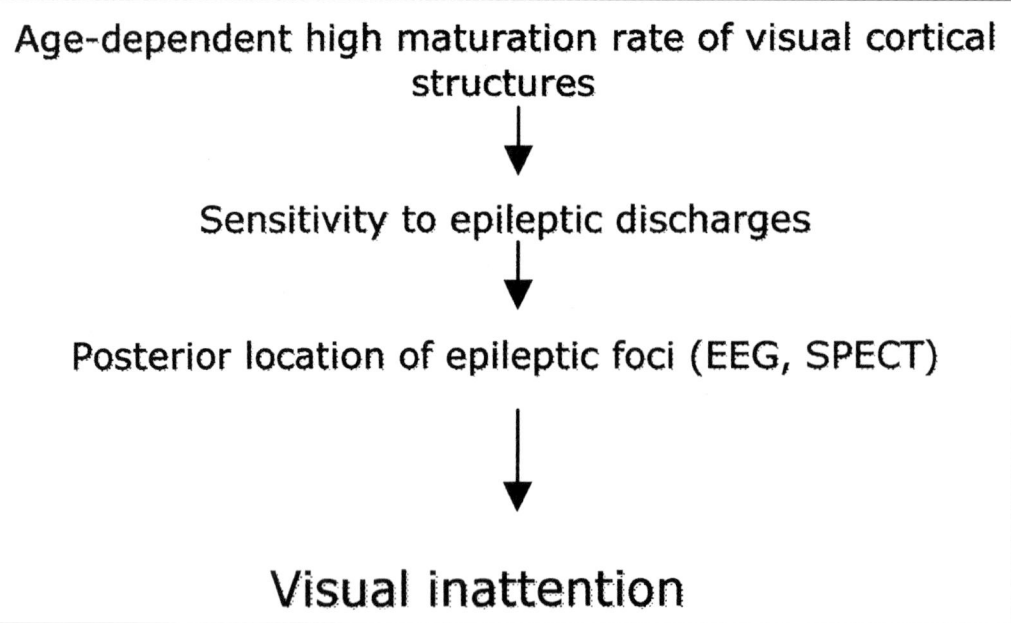

Figure 1. Cortical mechanism of visual attention in West syndrome.

presence of a central stimulus, the latter being possible only after the full maturation at around four months of the cortical control over the superior colliculus (Atkinson, 2000). This specific aspect of cortical maturation has been studied in infants with West syndrome in comparison with healthy controls and with a cohort of brain injured infants without epilepsy. The maturation of the fixation shift was definitely impaired in infants with West syndrome (*Figure 2*) in comparison with both control groups, representing a specific defect of visual function in this epileptic disorder.

This last finding strongly suggests that infantile spasms are associated with a high-level disorder of brain processing of visual stimuli. However, a possible impairment of the arousal system, mediated by the reticular formation, may also account for the disorder of visual behaviour (Guzzetta et al., 1993), as supported by the well known neuroradiological and neuropathological brain-stem changes in West syndrome (Chugani et al., 1992, Miyazaki et al., 1993; Satoh et al., 1986; Hayashi et al., 2000).

Similarly, at the spasm onset an impairment of the auditory function has been observed, concerning both a low-level and a high level disorder. In several studies an hypoacusia was sometimes detected in the acute stage of West syndrome with ABR audiometry (no V pic potential up to 80 dB), the site of the dysfunction being located at the level of, or beneath the, inferior colliculus (Kaga et al., 1982; Curatolo et al., 1989; Miyazaki et al., 1993; Baranello et al., 2006). As for the visual stimulus, an impairment of alertness may prevent auditory stimuli to be conveyed to the medial geniculate body up to the primary cortical auditory area. A low-level auditory impairment may thus occur in infants with West syndrome, suggesting a brain stem involvement as a possible mechanism for the auditory dysfunction (Kaga et al., 1982; Miyazaki et al., 1993). Conversely, some other studies have frequently found among the subjects with normal auditory threshold a lack of the ability to orient towards the acoustic stimulus, possibly due to a supracollicular dysfunction (Kaga et al., 1982; Baranello et al., 2006). Thus, a possibly high level auditory disorder may also be present at the onset of West syndrome. It occurs in auditory as well as visual stimulation even in cryptogenic forms, suggesting a responsibility of the epileptic disorder *per se*.

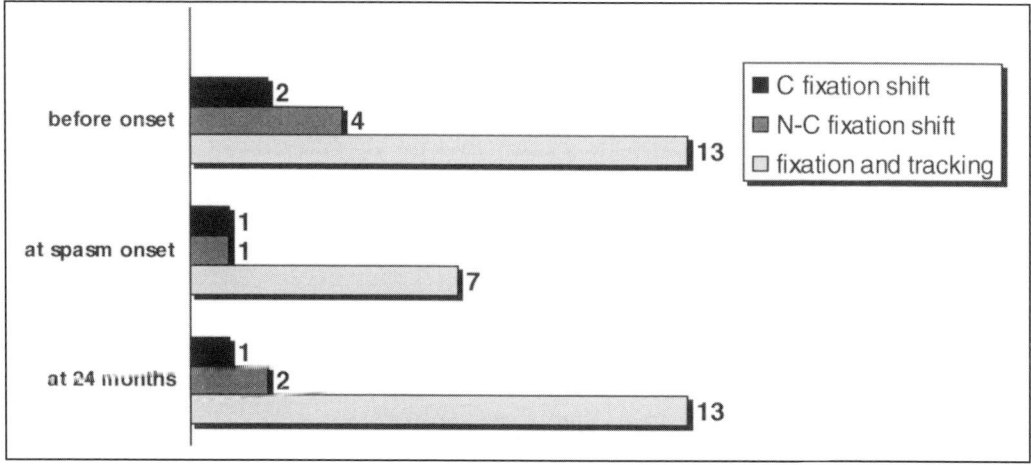

Figure 2. Evolution of visual attention in West syndrome.

Finally, somatosensiory evoked potentials too seem transiently involved in some cases of West syndrome (Shiroma *et al.*, 2004). So, multiple sensory functions appear to be impaired, especially during the first stages of the disease.

■ Disorders of cognitive development

Mental arrest or deterioration at the presentation of West syndrome has been described for several decades. The onset of the disease has generally been considered at the appearance of spasms, although we do not know if the real clinical beginning precedes the onset of spasms (see above). Mental impairment is usually more evident in cryptogenic forms, when no change of development occurs before the spasms onset, rather than in symptomatic forms, when early cognitive disorders can be explained by a primary underlying brain abnormality.

The developmental regression at the beginning of the disease consists of axial hypotonia, loss of reaching skills, poor smiling, and lack of responsiveness with a characteristic behavioural fluctuations of abilities. So far, the cognitive competence has rarely been assessed at the onset of spasms. Even in the more detailed studies, the results of cognitive competence examination during the acute stages of the disease generally do not come from a formal assessment with developmental scales (Jambaqué *et al.*, 1993, 2000; Vigevano *et al.*, 1993 ; Dulac *et al.*, 1986: 1993 ; Gaily *et al.*,1999; O'Callaghan *et al.*, 2004). Gaily *et al.* (1999), studying some cryptogenic forms, used the Muenchener Funktionelle Entwicklungsdiagnostik scale (MFED) (Hellbruegge *et al.*, 1985) but reported only little information concerning tracking and grasping: such skills were delayed in eight out of 15 infants and soon after cessation of spasms there was a delay in tracking and grasping in only six, four of them already delayed. In another study, a regression of vocal production at the onset of the syndrome has been reported (Jambaqué *et al.*, 1993).

The first analytical report of cognitive development in West syndrome concerns the Uzgiris-Hunt Scales performed in a cohort of 31 cases (Guzzetta *et al.*, 1993). These scales, aimed at specifically assessing cognitive abilities, showed that the most impaired skills were the permanence of objects, the vocal imitation and the operational causality. According to this study, the symptomatic forms, as expected, were generally delayed or strongly delayed, while infants with cryptogenic spasms had a better prognosis.

A more recent study using Griffiths' Scales showed at spasm onset a specific fall of competence at the Eye-Hand Coordination subscale, even in patients with otherwise normal range values (especially cryptogenic cases) (Randò *et al.*, 2005).

■ Developmental profiles

Profiles of cognitive evolution during the medium and long term follow-up of infants with West syndrome are variable *(Figure 3)* depending on multiple factors.

First of all, a benign evolution can certainly be observed, especially in cryptogenic spasms but also, although more rarely, in symptomatic cases (Vigevano *et al.*, 1993). In a retrospective study of infants with presumed cryptogenic West syndrome, Dulac *et al.* (1986) reported that lack of mental regression at the onset of spasms and absence of focal neurological and EEG abnormalities are positively associated with good prognosis. The favourable prognostic value of a normal developmental condition at onset (absence of deterioration of visual function such as eye tracking; lack of regression of some psychomotor skills) has been eventually confirmed by a subsequent prospective study (Dulac et al., 1993). The absence of interictal EEG foci and hypsarrhythmia between consecutive spasms (the so-called "non-independent" spasms) were according to the Dulac's group other features characterizing a possibly idiopathic form. Concurrently, another report stressed the presence among a series of cryptogenic cases of West of a presumably idiopathic form due to lack of "no known or suspected aetiology other than a possible hereditary predisposition" (Vigevano et al., 1993). The presence in a great part of infants with that form of a family history of other idiopathic epilepsies, or showing during the follow-up peculiar EEG genetic traits, confirmed the suspect of an idiopathic West syndrome. Indeed, the few patients named really "cryptogenjc", with poor prognosis, presented all at the end of the follow-up seizures, focal EEG abnormalities, and developmental delay "suggesting an underlying cerebral lesion". It is not easy, in such circumstances, to establish whether, or in which proportion, the evolution is related to the primary underlying cerebral lesion or to the effects of the epileptic disorder.

To asses the risk of cognitive impairment later in life in a group of infants with a benign form of cryptogenic West, Gaily et al. (1999) studied the cognitive development of 15 children whose spasms completely recovered within the first year of life. The assessment performed between the age of 4 and 5.9 years showed mild retardation in three children and normal global developmental quotient in the remaining twelve, but five of the latter group exhibited a specific cognitive deficit. So, eight children out of 15 had some cognitive problem.

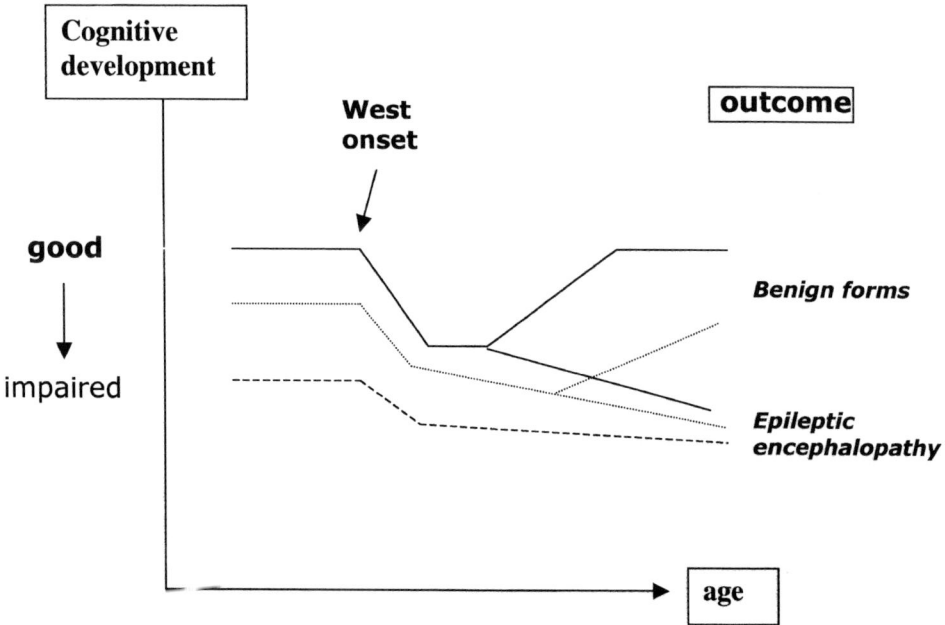

Figure 3. Profile of cognitive development in West syndrome.

Developmental condition at the age of 8 to 15 months after complete resolution of spasms seemed predictive of cognitive outcome. However, the lack of accurate systemic assessment before the age of 4 years raises some doubts on the normality of early development.

In a recent prospective multicentric study (Guzzetta et al., data not published) evaluating development in parallel with neurosensory assessment (visual and auditory) from spasm onset and for the following two years, cryptogenic patients showed a benign profile, for epilepsy and development. At onset, they generally presented with a global DQ within the normal range, even though with relatively poor results in hand and eye coordination scale in some, and with a frequent, although mild, sensory impairment concerning both cerebral visual and auditory functions (Randò et al., 2004, 2005; Baranello et al., 2006). For the same cohort, two years later, the evolution of epilepsy and of neurosensory and cognitive development was good; within six months after onset, epilepsy (hypsarrhythmia and seizures) recovered, the slight sensory impairment disappeared and cognitive development remained normal in all the infants. Therefore, neurosensory and cognitive impairment was mild and was paralleled by transient electroclinical abnormalities, and thoroughly recovered within six months from spasm onset. These results are consistent with what has been found by other investigators (Matsumoto et al., 1981; Bachman, 1982; Dulac et al., 1986, 1993; Vigevano et al., 1993). Moreover, in our study, the same profile was observed in three symptomatic patients, two of whom had tuberous sclerosis.

Several observations arise from our study: 1) it confirms the existence of a benign form of infantile spasms; 2) it shows, in this form, mild neurosensory and cognitive impairment at onset of spasms, that possibly makes these cases similar to the more severely affected patients with bad outcome; 3) a benign outcome does not concern exclusively the idiopathic forms, but also symptomatic cases whose brain lesions are still compatible with quite normal development; 4) initial good neurosensory and cognitive abilities represent a favourable prognostic factor.

The last prognostic consideration is not absolute because there are cases, extensively reported in the literature, that show progressive deterioration following an initially normal development. This is also confirmed by our prospective study that shows two cases with tuberous sclerosis presenting with normal development at the onset of spasms, and a subsequent gradual regression. Interestingly, the same cases were also characterized by persistent epileptic disorders (multifocal EEG abnormalities and partial seizures).

Our data confirm that West syndrome, at least in the deteriorating forms, deserves the definition of epileptic encephalopathy, "a condition in which the epileptiform abnormalities themselves are believed to contribute to the progressive disturbance in cerebral function" (Guerrini, 2006). The causative role of the epileptic disorder *per se* could be surely affirmed in cryptogenic forms that evolve towards developmental deterioration because of persistent epilepsy (non-benign forms). This is suggested by several reports, although brain structural or biochemical changes were not formally ruled out. Our more functionally detailed longitudinal study has not demonstrated progressive deterioration in cryptogenic patients. In non benign forms the presence of a brain injury makes it difficult to define the role of epilepsy in contributing "to the progressive disturbance in cerebral function".

In severely brain-injured infants that have severe developmental delay at spasm onset, brain lesions play a primary causative role; the responsibility of epilepsy in this clinical context remains minor. Different is the case of an initial mild or moderate delay; brain injury and the epileptic disorder interact in producing negative effects on developmental skills. The epileptic disorder prevents the re-organization of the functions that have been impaired by brain injury. In our quoted multicentric study, we observed that symptomatic cases with an initial cognitive delay could either show progressive deterioration or stable or mildly improved development. The former was associated with persistent severe epilepsy.

Developmental arrest or regression should not be considered as a necessary diagnostic element of West syndrome, as proposed by the West Delphi group (Lux and Osborne, 2005). The impairment of development can be mild and transitory in benign forms, either idiopathic or symptomatic, with good evolution; or may be stable although relevant in symptomatic forms without deterioration. When severe and progressive, these cases whether cryptogenic or symptomatic deserve to be defined as epileptic encephalopathies *(Figure 4)*.

This last hypothesis needs to be confirmed by prospective clinical and functional studies. Many additional variables should be investigated including aetiology and chronic administration of antiepileptic drugs.

Concerning long-term mental outcome, its relationship with initial evolution is difficult to analyze because many variables can intervene including drugs, habilitation and psychosocial factors (Guzzetta, 2006).

A) *Benign forms*

Cryptogenic (presumably idiopathic ?)

Symptomatic (compatible with normal development or mild/moderate retardation)

B) *Epileptic encephalopathy*

Cryptogenic deteriorating forms (presumably symptomatic ?)

Symptomatic deteriorating forms

Figure 4. Classification of West syndrome according to developmental evolution.

■ Neurosensory impairment and cognitive deterioration in West syndrome: a possible model

Maturation of neurosensory functions, and in particular visual function, is a gradual process during the first years of life. The early stages are acquired during the first months, spanning from the maturation of visual alertness to achievement of different aspects of visual attention. The infant is progressively able to integrate attention with the motor-spatial skills of reaching at and manipulating objects, up to the acquisition of the ability of moving (walking) through the environment at the end of the first year of life (Atkinson, 2000). A model based on information processing theories considers visual maturation a sort of pre-requisite for cognitive development. Visual behaviour indeed represents the general method to assess early cognitive competence. When representation and language abilities, as well as finalized motor schemes (praxias), are still absent, visual behaviour may indicate possible cognitive skills. However, other sensory channels, such as auditory pathways, can be involved in attention processes (Gomes *et al.* 2000), and both the visual and auditory modalities are generally considered to be the leading sensorial channels in early cognitive development (Posner and Petersen, 1990). This view explains why visual attention and, more in general, sensory and perceptual capabilities, have become the primary subjects of human cognitive neuroscience (Parasuraman 1998).

Attention seems strongly related to perceptual processing at this age. It might be hypothesised that the same neuronal circuits account for both attention and perceptual processing whatever model is considered; whether the "premotor" theory, according to which motor action modules are involved also in object analysis, or the "selection for action" theory, in which motor action is a function of sensory processing. Attentional performance is thus to be considered strictly correlated with good perceptual and learning abilities, and infant visual attention might be one of the best predictive factors of later cognitive capacity (Fagan, 1981; Fagan and Shepherd, 1987).

In this respect, it is not surprising that cognitive impairment and functional visual and auditory abnormalities, are closely linked in West syndrome. The pervasive epileptic disorder can prevent normal maturation of neural connectivity and, if persistent, impair cognitive development. Accordingly, in infants with West syndrome a tight relation can be found between the specific defect of early cognitive competence in the field of object permanence (Guzzetta *et al.*, 1993) and the impairment of visual function, since object permanence items are strongly dependent on visual skills, or between the low scores on the Eye-Hand Coordination subscale of the Griffiths' Scale and abnormal visual functions. It appears also consistent the relationship between the initial impairment of language development (items of vocal imitation in Uzgiris-Hunt Scales) and another relevant behavioural finding consisting of a disorder of interpersonal contact, sometimes evolving towards the autistic spectrum.

The study of the maturation of the visual function and of its disorders in the first months of life may thus represent a tool to understand possible deviations of the roots of cognition and to predict eventual cognitive delay (Atkinson, 2000). In early brain-injured infants, in fact, visual impairment seems related to disorders of neurodevelopment, confirming that visual function is strongly related to cognitive outcome (Cioni *et al.* 1996, Lanzi *et al.* 1998, Mercuri *et al.* 1999). There is evidence that in West syndrome visual and auditory functions are significantly related to cognitive development from the onset of spasms onset till two years later. The highly significant relationship that initially concerned neurosensory functions with in particular the scales linked with visual function (Griffiths' Eye & hand scale), eventually involved all the Griffiths' Scales suggesting a more pervasive effect of neurosensory impairment on cognitive competence (Randò *et al.*, 2004; Randò *et al.*o, 2005; Baranello *et al.*, 2006).

In some patients the onset of the visual and cognitive impairment that was independent from other possible causes such as brain lesions, was described even months before the appearance of spasms and hypsarrhythmia (Jambaqué, 1993; Guzzetta *et al.*, 2002), representing an early manifestation of epileptic encephalopathy. The possible prognostic value of this neuropsychological finding might be considered like other predictive neurophysiological signs reported in the literature (Watanabe *et al.*, 1987; Okumura and Watanabe, 2001), such as occipital discharges (Iinuma *et al.*, 1994).

The hypothesis of a direct correlation between early impairment of important sensorial channels and cognitive development is not contradictory with the cases of a congenital deficit of visual or auditory functions associated with a normal cognitive competence, nor with cases of brain pathology and mental delay without visual or auditory problems. On the one hand, the role of complex compensatory mechanisms, such as other neurosensory functions, may account for the achievement of a normal cognitive development in infants with impairment of the visual or auditory function. However, neurosensory functions alone cannot guarantee normal cognitive development if higher level functions are not spared. On the whole, the presence of multiple neurosensory disabilities and of a pervasive epileptic disorder preventing full brain re-organization, may be considered one of the most relevant causes of cognitive impairment in West syndrome. The specific epileptic disorder in West syndrome, eventually worsened by structural brain injuries involving eloquent cortical areas, seems to interfere with physiological functions in neural circuitries encompassing the visual and auditory domains, with consequent impairment of proper processing of sensory stimuli and of their higher integration. If the epileptic disorder subsides, sensory impairment is transitory; otherwise, functional re-organization is prevented and cognitive development itself is compromised resulting in progressive deterioration (*Figure 5*).

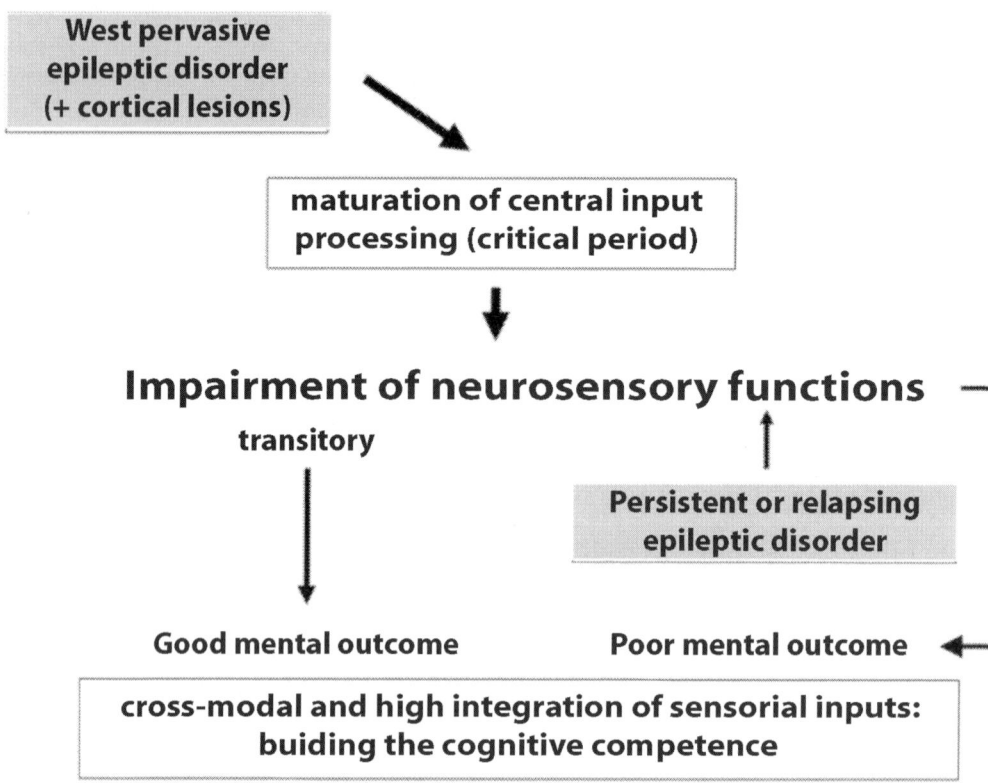

Figure 5. Mechanism of cognitive impairment in West syndrome: a possible model.

References

Atkinson J. *The developing visual brain*. Oxford, Oxford University Press, 2000.

Bachman DS. Use of valproic acid in treatment of infantile spasms. *Arch Neurol* 1982; 39: 49.52.

Baranello G, Randò T, Bancale A, et al. Auditory attention at the onset of West syndrome; correlation with EEG patterns and visual function. *Brain Dev* 2006; 28: 293-9.

Brooks BP, Simpson JL, Leber SM, Robertson PL, Archer SM. Infantile spasms as a cause of acquired perinatal visual loss. *JAAPOS* 2002; 6: 385-8.

Castano G, Lyons CJ, Jan JE, Connolly M. Cortical visual impairment in children with infantile spasms. *JAAPOS* 2000; 4: 175-8.

Cioni G, Fazzi B, Ipata A, Canapicchi R, van Hoof-van Duin J Correlation between cerebral visual impairment and magnetic resonance imaging in children with neonatal encephalopathy. *Dev Med Child Neurol* 1996; 38: 120-32.

Curatolo P, Cardona F, Cusmai R. BAEPs in infantile spasms. *Brain Dev* 1989; 1: 347-8.

Chugani HT, Shields WD, Shewmon DA, Olson DM, Phelps ME, Peacock WJ. Infantile spasms : PET identifies focal cortical dysgenesis in cryptogenic cases for surgical treatment. *Ann Neurol* 1990; 27: 406-13.

Chugani HT, Shewmon DA, Sankar R, Chen BC, Phelps ME. Infantile spasms: lenticular nuclei and brain stem activation on positron emission tomography. *Ann Neurol* 1992; 31: 212-9.

Chugani HT, Shewmon DA, Shields WD, et al. Surgery for intractable infantile spasms: neuroimaging perspective. *Epilepsia* 1993; 34: 764-71.

Commission on Pediatric Epilepsy of the International League Against Epilepsy. Workshp on infantile spasms. *Epilepsia* 1992; 33: 195.

Dongier S, Charles C, Chabert F. Séméiologie psychiatrique et psychométrique... In: Gastaut H, *(syndrome de West)*. Paris, Masson 1964: 53-64.

Dulac O, Plouin P, Jambaque I, Motte J. Spasmes infantiles épileptiques bénins. *Rev Electroencephalogr Neurophysiol Clin* 1986; 16: 371-82.

Dulac O, Plouin P, Jambaque I. Predicting favourable outcome in idiopathic West syndrome. *Epilepsia* 1993; 34: 747-56.

Fagan JF. The relationship of novelty preference during infancy to later intelligence and recognition memory. *Intelligence* 1981; 8: 339-46.

Fagan JF, Shepherd PA *The Fagan Test of infant intelligence training manual*. Vol. 4, Cleveland, Infantest Corporation, 1987.

Gaily E, Appelqvist K, Kantola-Sorsa E, et al. Cognitive deficits after cryptogenic infantile spasms with benign seizure evolution. *Dev Med Child Neurol* 1999; 41: 660-4.

Gomes H, Malholm S, Christodoulou C, Ritter W, Cowan N The development of auditory attention. *Frontiers in Bioscience* 2000; 5: 108-20.

Guerrini R. Epilepsy in children. *Lancet* 2006; 367: 499-524.

Guzzetta F. Cognitive and behavioural outcome of epileptic syndromes: West syndrome. *Epilepsia* 2006; 47 (suppl 2): 49-52.

Guzzetta F, Crisafulli A, Isaya Crinò M. Cognitive assessment of infants with West syndrome: how useful is it for diagnosis and prognosis? *Dev Med Child Neurol* 1993; 35: 379-87.

Guzzetta F, Frisone MF, Ricci D, Rando' T, Guzzetta A. Development of visual attention in West syndrome. *Epilepsia* 2002; 43: 757-63.

Hayashi M, Itoh M, Araki S, et al. Immunohistochemical analysis of brainstem lesions in infantile spasms. *Neuropathology* 2000; 20: 297-303.

Hellbruegge T, Lajosi F, Menara D, Shanberger R, Rautenstrauch T. *Muenchener Funktionelle Entwicklungsdiagnostik*. Luebeck, HansischesVerlagkontor, 1985.

Iinuma K, Haginoya K, Nagai M, Kon K, Yagi T, Saito T. Visual abnormalities and occipital EEG discharges: risk factors for West syndrome. *Epilepsia* 1994; 35: 806-9.

Illingsworth RS. Sudden mental deterioration with convulsions in infancy. *Arch Dis Child* 1955; 30: 529-37.

Jambaqué I, Chiron C, Dulac O, Raynaud C, Syrota P. Visual inattention in West syndrome: a neuropsychological and neurofunctional imaging study. *Epilepsia* 1993; 34: 692-700.

Jambaqué I, Chiron C, Dumas C, Munford J, Dulac O. Mental and behavioural outcome of infantile epilepsy treated by vigabatrin in tuberous sclerosis patients. *Epilepsy Res* 2000; 38: 151-60.

Kaga K, Marsh RR, Fukuyama Y. Auditory brain stem responses in infantile spasms. *Inter J Ped Otorhinolar* 1982; 4: 57-67.

Koo B, Hwang P. Localization of focal cortical lesions influences age of onset of infantile spasms. *Epilepsia* 1996; 37: 1068-71.

Lanzi G, Fazzi E, Uggetti C, Cavallini A, Danova S, Egitto MG. Cerebral visual impairment in periventricular leukomalacia. *Neuropediatrics* 1998; 29: 145-50.

Lux AI, Osborne P. A proposal for case definitions and outcome measures in studies of infantile spasms and West syndrome: consensus statement of the West Delphi group. *Epilepsia* 2004; 45: 1416-28.

Matsumoto A, Watanabe K, Negoro T, et al. Infantile spasms: etiological factors, clinical aspects, and long-term prognosis in 200 cases. *Eur J Pediatr* 1981; 135: 239-44.

Mercuri E, Haataja L, Guzzetta A, Anker S, Cowan F, Rutherford M. Visual function in term infants with hypoxic-ischaemic insults: correlation with neurodevelopment at 2 years of age. *Arch Dis Child Fetal Neonatal Ed* 1999; 80: F99-F104.

Miyzaki M, Hashimoto T, Tayama M, Kuroda Y. Brainstem involvement in infantile spasms: a study emplying brainstem evoked potentials and magnetic resonance imaging. *Neuropediatrics* 1993; 24: 126-30.

O'Callaghan FJ, Harris T, Joinson C, et al. The relation of infantile spasms, tubers, and intelligence in tuberous sclerosis complex. *Arch Dis Child* 2004; 89: 530-3.

Okumura A, Watanabe K. Clinico-electrical evolution in pre-hypsarrhythmic stage: towards prediction and prevention of West syndrome. *Brain Dev* 2001; 23: 482-7.

Parasuraman R. The attentive brain issues and prospects. In. Parasuraman R (ed) *The attentive brain*. Cambridge, MA, MIT Press, 1998;. 3-15.

Posner MA, Petersen SE. The attention system of the human brain. *Ann Rev Neurosci* 1990; 13: 25-42.

Randò T, Bancale A, Baranello G, et al. Visual function in infants with West syndrome: correlation with EEG patterns. *Epilepsia* 2004; 45: 781-6.

Randò T, Bancale A, Baranello G, et al. Cognitive competence at the onset of West sindrome: correlation with EEG-patterns and visual function. *Dev Med Child Neurol* 2005; 47: 760-5.

Satoh J, Mizurani T, Morimatsu Y. Neuropsthology of brainstem in age-dependent epileptic encephalopathy, especially of cases with infantile spasms. *Brain Dev* 1986; 8: 443-9.

Shiroma N, Fukumizu M, Sugai K, Sasaki M, Kaga M. Serial median nerve SEPs and SSEPs in patients with West syndrome. *No To Hattatsu* 2004; 36: 45-8.

Suzuki M, Okumura A, Watanabe K, et al. The predictive value of electroencephalogram durino early infancy for later development of West sindrome in infants with cystic periventricular leukomalacia. *Epilepsia* 2003; 44: 443-6.

Taddeucci G, Fiorentini A, Pirchio M, Spinelli D. Abnormal pattern reversal evoked potentials. *Human Neurobiol* 1984; 3: 153-155.

Vigevano F, Fusco L, Cusmai R, Claps D, Ricci S, Milani L. The idiopathic form of West syndrome. *Epilepsia*. 1993; 34: 743-76.

Watanabe K, Takeuchi I, Hakamada S, Hayakawa F. Neurophysiological and neuroradiological features preceding spasms. *Brain Dev* 1987; 9: 391-8.

Wenzel D. Abnormal VEP and SEP: functional "blindness". *Brain Dev* 1987; 9: 365-8.

Surgical treatment of West syndrome

Harry T Chugani[1,2,3], **Eishi Asano**[1,2], **Sandeep Sood**[4]

[1] *Carman and Ann Adams Department of Pediatrics*
[2] *Departments of Neurology*
[3] *Radiology*
[4] *Neurosurgery*
Children's Hospital of Michigan, Wayne State University, Detroit, Michigan, USA

The increase in surgical treatment of West syndrome in the past two decades is directly linked to rapid advances in both anatomical and functional neuroimaging (Chugani & Pinard, 1994). These advances, together with detailed analysis of EEG activity, including the use of quantitative EEG analysis, have also led to an evolution from prior concepts of infantile spasms as primary generalized seizures to the current thinking that infantile spasms have a *focal* onset with a pattern of secondary generalization that is age-specific. In this chapter, we begin with a brief account of the history of surgery for West syndrome and then review the growing literature to support a role for epilepsy surgery in *selected* cases of intractable infantile spasms.

■ History of surgical treatment in West syndrome

The observation in several case reports that surgical removal of focal structural brain lesions in patients with infantile spasms led to cessation of the spasms was intriguing and suggested that these lesions were involved somehow in the generation of the spasms. One of the earliest cases was a 7-month-old infant who, following removal of a choroid plexus papilloma, became seizure free and at one year follow up was developing normally (Branch and Dyken, 1979). Another child, with infantile spasms and a right temporal lobe astrocytoma, became seizure free following resection of the tumor (Mimaki *et al.*, 1983) and, subsequently, a number of other cases were reported where resection of a focal lesion led to cessation of infantile spasms (*e.g.*, Ogata *et al.*, 1985; Ruggieri *et al.*, 1989; Uthman *et al.*, 1991). The first reported *series* consisted of 10 patients with infantile spasms and porencephalic cysts in whom neurosurgical marsupalization of the cysts and fenestration to the ventricular system resulted in resolution of the infantile spasms (Palm *et al.*, 1988).

The observation that positron emission tomography (PET) of glucose metabolism could identify focal cortical abnormalities corresponding to epileptogenic regions in patients with *cryptogenic* infantile spasms *(Figure 1)* and that these infants could benefit from cortical resection (Chugani et al., 1990) was initially met with a great deal of skepticism (Hrachovy et al., 1991). However, even before this, French investigators had already found evidence of focal hypoperfusion using single photon emission computed tomography (SPECT) in patients with West syndrome and normal CT scans (Dulac et al., 1987). Since MRI scans were not performed on these subjects, a small or subtle lesion could not be ruled out, as demonstrated subsequently by the same authors who found MRI lesions in West syndrome patients with normal CT scans (van Bogaert et al., 1993). The locations of both anatomical and functional focal abnormalities tended to favor the parieto-temporo-occipital areas (Dulac et al., 1987; Cusmai et al., 1988; Chugani et al., 1990). In general, more posteriorly located foci are associated with earlier onset of spasms, whereas frontal lobe foci are less common and tend to be associated with later onset of spasms (Koo & Hwang, 1996), in agreement with the rank order of functional maturation for these cortical regions (Chugani et al., 1987).

Although the typical findings on functional neuroimaging consist of focal hypometabolism (Chugani et al., 1990; 1993; Fois et al., 1995; Ferrie et al., 1996) or hypoperfusion (Dulac et al., 1987; Cusmai et al., 1988; Miyazaki et al., 1994), increased glucose metabolism or blood flow may also be occasionally seen (Chugani et al., 1993; Chiron et al., 1993; Kumada et al., 2006). Furthermore, some investigators (Maeda et al., 1993) have reported that the focal cortical hypometabolism shown on PET scans may be transient with total recovery after cessation of spasms suggesting that the PET abnormality may be purely on a functional basis, although the presence of a small or subtle structural abnormality cannot be ruled out. Indeed, when focal resections are performed on cortical areas showing abnormal metabolism or perfusion on PET or SPECT, neuropathological examination of the resected tissue typically reveals cortical dysplasia (Chugani et al., 1990; Vinters et al., 1992; Chugani et al., 1993; Asano et al., 2001).

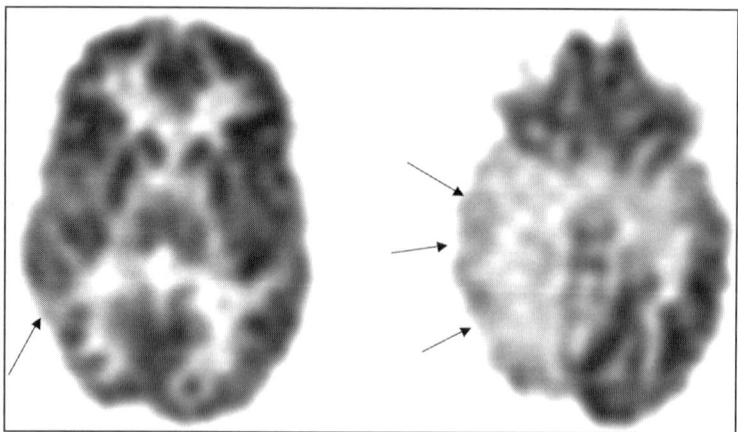

Figure 1. Positron Emission Tomography (PET) identifying epileptic regions in a patient with cryptogenic infantile spasms.

Despite the previous controversy as to whether it is appropriate to perform surgery for infantile spasms (Hrachovy et al., 1991), surgical resection of focal cortical regions guided in part by anatomical or functional neuroimaging is now widely accepted and carried in many centers worldwide (Holmes, 1993; Wyllie et al., 1996; Hwang et al., 1996; Kramer et al., 1997; Saneto & Wyllie, 2000; Hoffman, 2002), even in infants younger than 6 months of age (Kang et al., 2006). The early series of Chugani et al. (1993) consisted of 23 patients with infantile spasms who underwent cortical resection (n = 15) or hemispherectomy (n = 8). Infantile spasms were present at the time of surgery in 17 of the 23 children, whereas there had been a recent evolution to other seizure types in 6 subjects. Interestingly, PET was the only imaging modality to identify a cortical focus in 14 of the 23 patients. The results were excellent with 15 children achieving total seizure freedom, 3 with 90% seizure control and one with 75% seizure control. In a subsequent analysis of a large series of 140 patients with infantile spasms it was demonstrated that, with the benefit of PET scanning, the number of symptomatic cases rose dramatically from 42 (30.0%) to 134 (95.7%). The majority of abnormalities detected on PET were unifocal or multifocal hypometabolic areas presumably representing dysplastic lesions (Chugani & Conti, 1996).

■ Presurgical evaluation

When infantile spasms remain resistant to first-line treatments such as vigabatrin, ACTH and zonisamide, potential surgical approaches should be considered. Usually, by this time, the more obvious non-surgical cases would have already been recognized, such as various metabolic disorders, chromosomal abnormalities, diffuse brain injuries and diffuse brain malformations. Focal EEG findings suggest that there may be an underlying structural substrate responsible for triggering the spasms. However, when hypsarrhythmia is present on the EEG, focal electrographic abnormalities may be difficult to detect and, therefore, EEG recordings either preceding or following the presence of hypsarrhythmia should be carefully analyzed for focal features. The most revealing instances are when partial seizures evolve directly into, or are associated with, a cluster of spasms (Dalla Bernardina et al., 1984; Yamamoto et al., 1988; Donat & Wright, 1991; Carrazana et al., 1993; Gaily et al., 1995). In some cases, the intracranial EEG reveals a leading spike which we have found to be a useful marker for the trigger zone for the spasms (Asano et al., 2005) (Figure 2).

When the MRI scan shows a unilateral structural abnormality and there is good concordance with the ictal EEG, it can be argued that PET scanning is not necessary. However, we have found that even in such cases, glucose metabolism PET studies provide important complementary information. For example, the extent of the epileptogenic or "nociferous" cortex is typically underestimated by the MRI and a lesionectomy may be insufficient to achieve an optimum seizure and developmental outcome. The extent of functional disturbances on PET serves as a useful guide for subdural electrode placements to ensure a more comprehensive evaluation of potential epileptogenic zones. Furthermore, contralateral "silent" abnormalities may be detected with PET and their presence would have important prognostic significance suggesting a less favorable cognitive outcome even if the seizures can be controlled with a resection. One should be cautious in interpreting MRI scans if these are

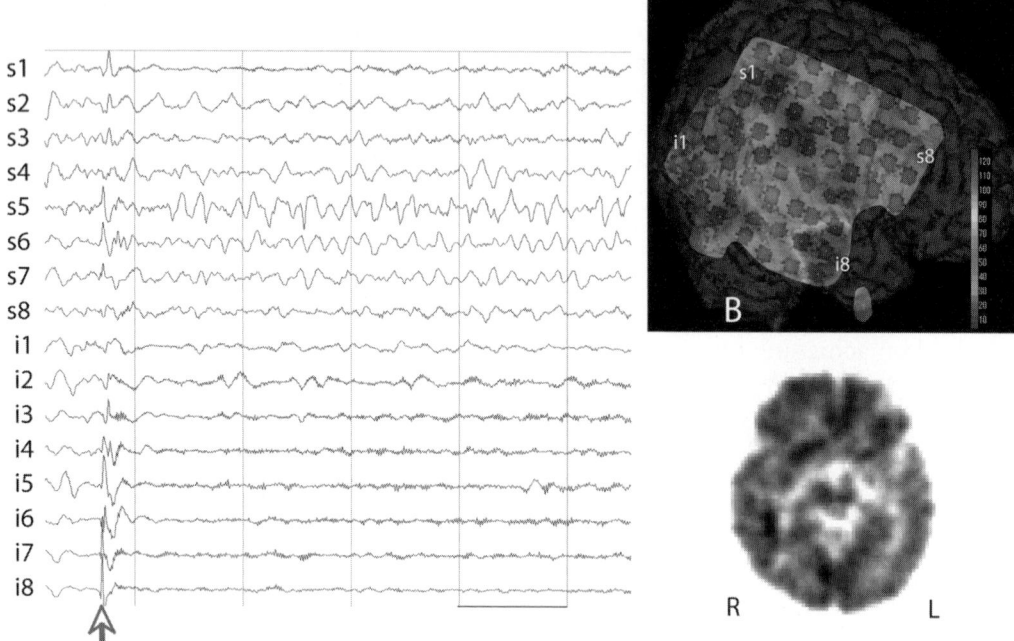

Figure 2. Infantile spasms associated with cortical dysplasia in the right temporal lobe.

performed in the first year of life at the presentation of West syndrome, since poor grey-white matter differentiation may not yet be obvious but may become quite apparent later in the second or third years (Sankar et al., 1995).

We suggest that all patients with cryptogenic infantile spasms resistant to conventional medical treatment should have a PET scan of glucose metabolism. Four different types of abnormalities have been observed in these children (Figure 3). When a single region of abnormal glucose metabolism is present, and there is good concordance with the focus identified on the EEG, surgical removal of the epileptogenic region results not only in seizure control but also in complete or partial reversal of the associated developmental delay. Unfortunately, about 65% of infants with cryptogenic spasms show more than one area of cortical hypometabolism on the PET scan (Chugani & Conti, 1996) and are therefore not ideal candidates for cortical resection. We have, on occasion, performed a "palliative" cortical resection in some of these children with very severe epilepsy in order to improve their quality of life provided that the majority of their seizures arise from one focus. However, even if their seizures are abolished, these children usually may not benefit significantly in terms of cognitive improvement from the "palliative" resection, and this must be clearly explained to the parents prior to surgery.

About 10% of all infants with cryptogenic spasms will show bilateral temporal lobe hypometabolism on their PET scans (Figure 3). These children show a distinct clinical phenotype characterized by severe developmental delay (particularly in the language domain) and autism (Chugani et al., 1996). The PET scan may reveal, in some cases,

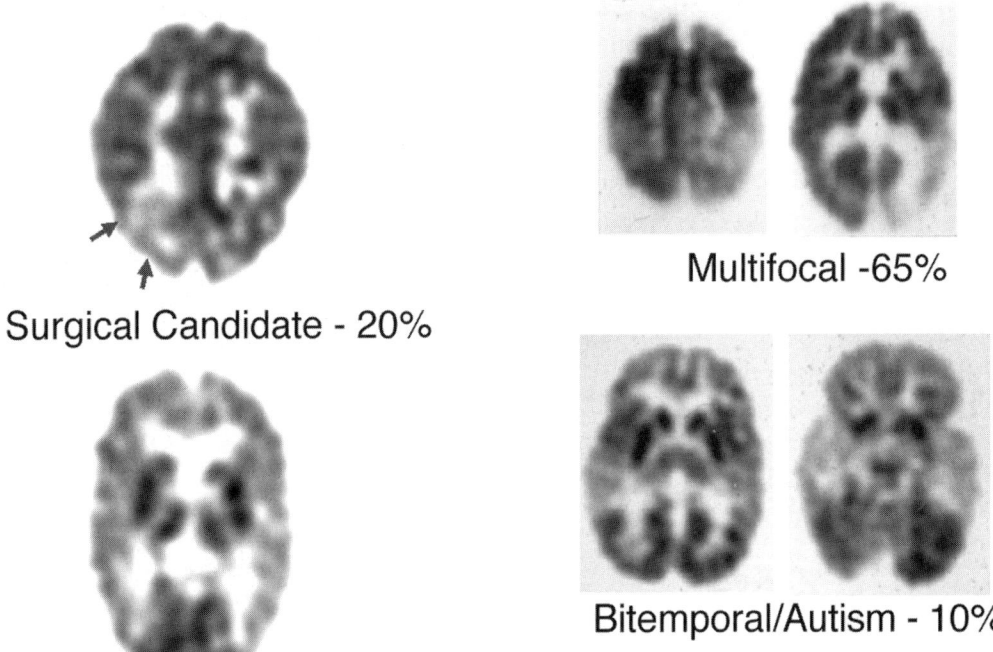

Figure 3. Infantile spasms: metabolic patterns.

bilateral symmetric or generalized cortical hypometabolism, with or without associated cerebellar involvement *(Figure 3)*. This type of pattern is not suggestive of an underlying lesional etiology but, rather, may indicate an underlying genetic/metabolic condition. When this pattern is encountered, more detailed metabolic and genetic studies should be performed and the idea of cortical resection should be abandoned. Finally, it is important to point out that since the ketogenic diet does not allow for glucose metabolism in the brain to proceed in a normal manner, the PET scan should not be performed when the child is on this diet as the results are difficult to interpret.

■ Tuberous sclerosis

One of the more common symptomatic causes of infantile spasms for which surgical resection may be highly beneficial is tuberous sclerosis. However, to pinpoint the epileptogenic tuber amidst a multitude of tubers can be very challenging. In some instances, the ictal EEG may disclose very clearly the general epileptogenic zone so that liberal coverage with intracranial electrodes will adequately sample the epileptic focus. Unfortunately, localization or even lateralization of the seizure focus is often very difficult and potential surgery for refractory seizures is not further pursued based on EEG findings. For example, an epileptogenic tuberous region situated in medial brain regions may not reveal lateralized seizure onset on the EEG, but may show a generalized pattern of epileptic discharges.

Neuroimaging with MRI, glucose metabolism PET and even flumazenil PET is not able to differentiate between epileptogenic and non-epileptogenic tubers. Although ictal SPECT may occasionally highlight the epileptogenic tuber, the seizures in these children are often quite brief and an ictal study is difficult to achieve without several attempts. We have developed PET scanning with alpha-[^{11}C]methyl-L-tryptophan (AMT) as a very approach to pinpoint the epileptogenic tuberous region in patients whose seizures are uncontrolled and surgery is being considered (Chugani et al., 1988; Asano et al., 2000). Because AMT (an analogue of tryptophan) accumulates in the vicinity of the seizure focus, PET scanning of this radiotracer reveals an *increased* signal in the *interictal* state. This feature of AMT makes it an ideal PET tracer in patients with multiple lesions, not all of which may be epileptogenic *(Figure 4)*.

In our surgical series, the AMT PET approach was used in the preoperative evaluation of 17 children (mean age: 4.7 years) with TSC and intractable epilepsy (Kagawa et al., 2005). Fourteen of the 17 children had long-term intracranial EEG monitoring. Increased AMT uptake was found in 30 tubers of 16 patients and 23 of these tubers (77%) were located in epileptic foci as defined by intracranial EEG. In 3 of the 17 children, a "palliative" surgery was performed because an optimal resection would have resulted in unacceptable consequences such as hemiplegia. Of the remaining 14 patients, 12 became seizure-free. There was an excellent correlation between resection of tubers showing increased AMT uptake and good outcome (Kagawa et al., 2005; see Roach, 2005 for editorial).

Although clearly an advance in seizure focus localization in patients with TSC, cortical areas of increased AMT uptake are seen in only about 2/3 of subjects. The remaining patients, while their seizures are poorly controlled with medications, fail to show any areas of increased AMT uptake. It is not clear why this is the case, but the fact that it is possible to differentiate epileptic from non-epileptic tubers using an interictal neuroimaging tool is a strong impetus to pursue aggressively other potential PET tracers for this purpose.

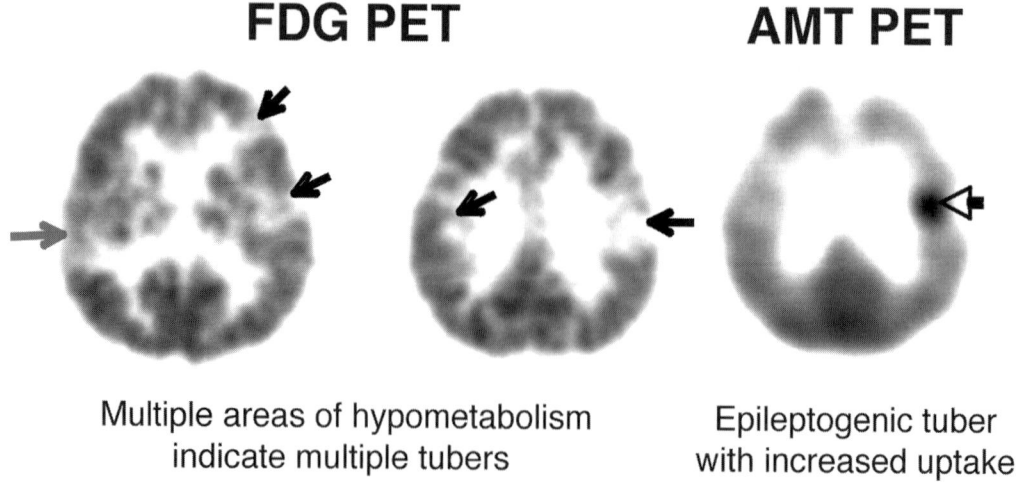

Figure 4. AMT PET in Tuberous Sclerosis identifies epileptogenic lesion(s).

Corpus callosotomy

There have been very few cases reported on corpus callosotomy as a treatment for refractory infantile spasms. In one report on two children with West syndrome, the spasms became asymmetric and the hypsarrhythmia unilateral following corpus callosotomy (Pinard et al., 1993). This suggested that the corpus callosum is important for the generalization of hypsarrhythmia. In their series on epileptic spasms beyond infancy, Talwar et al. (1995) indicated that 2 of 3 patients experienced a marked reduction in seizure frequency after corpus callosotomy by parental report, although post-operative video-EEG monitoring was not performed. The French group (Pinard et al., 1999) later reported their results on corpus callosotomy in 17 children with symptomatic generalized epilepsy *after* West syndrome. They found that, after complete callosotomy, spasms disappeared in 80% of children and drop attacks completely stopped or were dramatically reduced in 90% of children. In 9 children, there was an improvement in cognitive function and behavior. It is safe to say that while some patients with infantile spasms may have benefited from corpus callosotomy, more studies are needed to assess the potential benefit of callosotomy in this patient group.

References

Asano E, Chugani DC, Muzik O et al. Multimodality imaging for improved detection of epileptogenic lesions in children with tuberous sclerosis complex. *Neurology* 2000; 54: 1976-84.

Asano E, Chugani DC, Juhász C, Muzik O, Chugani HT. Surgical treatment of West syndrome. *Brain Dev* 2001; 23: 668-76.

Asano E, Juhasz C, Shah A et al. Origin and propagation of epileptic spasms delineated on electrocorticography. *Epilepsia* 2005; 46: 1087-97.

Branch CE, Dyken PR. Choroid plexus papilloma and infantile spasms. *Ann Neurol* 1979; 5: 302-4.

Carrazana EJ, Lombroso CT, Mikati M, Helmers S, Holmes GL. Facilitation of infantile spasms by partial seizures. *Epilepsia* 1993; 34: 97-109.

Chiron C, Dulac O, Bulteau C et al. Study of regional cerebral blood flow in West syndrome. *Epilepsia* 1993; 34: 707-15.

Chugani DC, Chugani HT, Muzik O et al. Imaging epileptogenic tubers in children with tuberous sclerosis complex using alpha-[^{11}C]methyl-L-tryptophan positron emission tomography. *Ann Neurol* 1998; 44: 858-66.

Chugani HT, Phelps ME, Mazziotta JC. Positron emission tomography study of human brain functional development. *Ann Neurol* 1987; 22: 487-97.

Chugani HT, Shields WD, Shewmon DA, Olson DM, Phelps ME, Peacock WJ. Infantile spasms: I. PET identifies focal cortical dysgenesis in cryptogenic cases for surgical treatment. *Ann Neurol* 1990; 27: 406-13.

Chugani HT, Shewmon DA, Shields WD et al. Surgery for intractable infantile spasms: neuroimaging perspectives. *Epilepsia* 1993; 34: 764-71.

Chugani HT, Pinard JM. Surgical treatment. In Dulac O, Chugani HT, Dalla Bernardina B (eds.): *Infantile Spasms and West Syndrome*. Saunders, London, 1994: 257-66.

Chugani HT, Conti JR. Etiologic classification of infantile spasms in 140 cases: role of positron emission tomography. *J Child Neurol* 1996; 11: 44-8.

Chugani HT, Da Silva E, Chugani DC. Infantile spasms: III. Prognostic implications of bitemporal hypometabolism on positron emission tomography. *Ann Neurol* 1996; 39: 643-9.

Cusmai R, Dulac O, Diebler C. Lésions focales dans les spasmes infantiles. *Neurophysiol Clin* 1988; 18: 235-41.

Dalla Bernardina, B., Colamaria, V., Capovilla, G. Sindromi epilettiche precoci e malformazioni cerebrali: studio multicentrico. *Bollettino – Lega Italiana contro l'Epilessia* 1984; 45-46: 65-7.

Donat JF, Wright FS. Simultaneous infantile spasms and partial seizures. *J Child Neurol* 1991; 6: 246-50.

Dulac O, Raynaud C, Chiron C, Plouin P, Syrota A, Arthuis M. Étude du débit sanguin cérébral dans le syndrome de West idiopathique: corrélation avec les données électroencéphalographiques. *Rev EEG Neurophysiol Clin* 1987; 17: 169-82.

Ferrie CD, Maisey M, Cox T, Polkey C et al. Focal abnormalities detected by 18FDG PET in epileptic encephalopathies. *Arch Dis Child* 1996; 75: 102-7.

Fois A, Farnetani MA, Balestri P et al. EEG, PET, SPET and MRI in intractable childhood epilepsies: possible surgical correlations. *Childs Nerv Syst* 1995; 11: 672-8.

Gaily EK, Shewmon DA, Chugani HT, Curran JG. Asymmetric and asynchronous infantile spasms. *Epilepsia* 1995; 36: 873-82.

Hoffman HJ. Surgery for West's syndrome. *Adv Exp Med Biol* 2002; 497: 57-9.

Holmes GL. Surgery for intractable seizures in infancy and early childhood. *Neurology* 1993; 43 (suppl 5): S28-S37.

Hrachovy RA, Frost JD Jr, Glaze DG, Kellaway P. Surgical treatment for infantile spasms? *Ann Neurol* 1991; 29: 110-2.

Hwang PA, Otsubo H, Koo BKK et al. Infantile spasms: cerebral blood flow abnormalities correlate with EEG, neuroimaging, and pathologic findings. *Pediatr Neurol* 1996; 14: 220-5.

Kagawa K, Chugani DC, Asano E et al. Epilepsy surgery outcome in children with tuberous sclerosis complex evaluated with alpha-[11C]methyl-L-tryptophan positron emission tomography (PET). *J Child Neurol* 2005; 20: 429-38.

Kang HC, Jung DE, Kim KM, Hwang YS, Park SK, Ko TS. Surgical treatment of two patients with infantile spasms in early infancy. *Brain Dev* 2006, in press.

Koo B, Hwang P. Localization of focal cortical lesions influences age of onset of infantile spasms. *Epilepsia* 1996; 37: 1068-71.

Kramer U, Whey-Chen S, Mikati MA. Focal features in West syndrome indicating candidacy for surgery. *Pediatr Neurol* 1997; 16: 213-7.

Kumada T, Okazawa H, Yamauchi H, Kitoh T, Ito M. Focal glucose hepermetabolism in interictal state of West syndrome. *Pediatr Neurol* 2006; 34: 47-50.

Maeda N, Watanabe K, Negoro T et al. Transient focal cortical hypometabolism in idiopathic West syndrome. *Pediatr Neurol* 1993; 9: 430-4.

Mimaki T, Ono J, Yabuuchi H. Temporal lobe astrocytoma with infantile spasms. *Ann Neurol* 1983; 14: 695-6.

Miyazaki M, Hashimoto T, Fujii E, Tayama M, Kuroda Y. Infantile spasms: localized cerebral lesions on SPECT. *Epilepsia* 1994; 35: 988-92.

Ogata H, Mitsudome A, Yokota K, Tachibana H. Three cases of infantile spasms with brain cystic lesions. *Brain Dev* 1985; 7: 184.

Palm DG, Brandt M, Korinthenberg R. West syndrome and Lennox-Gastaut syndrome in children with porencephalic cysts: long-term follow-up after neurosurgical treatment. In: Niedermeyer E, Degen R, eds. *The Lennox-Gastaut syndrome*. New York: Alan R. Liss, 1988: 419-26.

Pinard JM, Delalande O, Plouin P, Dulac O. Callosotomy in West syndrome suggests a cortical origin of hypsarrhythmia. *Epilepsia* 1993; 34: 780-7.

Pinard JM, Delalande O, Chiron C et al. Callosotomy for epilepsy after West syndrome. *Epilepsia* 1999; 40: 1727-34.

Roach ES. Seeing with new eyes: using positron emission tomography (PET) to identify epileptogenic tubers. *J Child Neurol* 2005; 20: 399.

Ruggieri V, Caraballo R, Fejerman N. Intracranial tumors and West syndrome. *Pediatr Neurol* 1989; 5: 327-9.

Saneto RP, Wyllie E. Epilepsy surgery in infancy. *Semin Pediatr Neurol* 2000; 7: 187-93.

Sankar R, Curran JG, Kevill JW, Rintahaka PJ, Shewmon DA, Vinters HV. Microscopic cortical dysplasia in infantile spasms: evolution of white matter abnormalities. *Am J Neuroradiol* 1995; 16: 1265-72.

Talwar D, Baldwin MA, Hutzler R, Griesemer DA. Epileptic spasms in older children: persistence beyond infancy. *Epilepsia* 1995; 36: 151-5.

Uthman BM, Reid SA, Wilder BJ, Andriola MR, Beydoun AA. Outcome for West syndrome following surgical treatment. *Epilepsia* 1991; 32: 668-71.

Van Bogaert P, Chiron C, Adamsbaum C, Robain O, Diebler C, Dulac O. Value of magnetic resonance imaging in West syndrome of unknown etiology. *Epilepsia* 1993; 34: 701-6.

Vinters HV, Fisher RS, Cornford ME *et al*. Morphological substrates of infantile spasms: studies based on surgically resected cerebral tissue. *Childs Nerv Syst* 1992; 8: 8-17.

Wyllie E, Comair YG, Kotagal P, Raja S, Ruggieri P. Epilepsy surgery in infants. *Epilepsia* 1996; 37: 625-37.

Yamamoto N, Watanabe K, Negoro T *et al*. Partial seizures evolving to infantile spasms. *Epilepsia* 1988; 29: 34-40.

The medical treatment of infantile spasms

Giangennaro Coppola, Antonio Pascotto

Clinic of Child Neuropsychiatry, Second University of Naples, Italy

The treatment of infantile spasms is still surrounded by a thick fog, probably due to the incomplete knowledge of the physiopathological mechanisms of the spasms. Such uncertainty is witnessed by the following words by Baram (2003): "Over 150 years after the description of infantile spasms, fifty years after the delineation of hypsarrhythmia, and forty years after the coining of the term "West syndrome", there is little progress in understanding and effectively treating this disorder".

An officially approved therapy for infantile spasms has yet to be approved by FDA. A limited number of randomised controlled trials of drugs considered to be the most effective therapies for IS, *e.g.* ACTH/corticosteroids and vigabatrin, are presently available for review. These studies are of limited value because of an often small number of patients included, by markedly different methodologies including the kind of drug (*e.g.* natural or synthetic ACTH), the daily dose, the duration of treatment, the criteria for assessing the treatment effectiveness, mostly limited to spasm cessation, thereby the results are inconclusive.

Studies on the therapy of infantile spasms are generally difficult to carry on, as they often require a multicenter network to get a significant number of patients; furthermore, long-term studies are even more difficult, because of the difficulty to maintain the enrolled patients into the study.

Some of the criteria that should help choosing a given treatment option are: 1) the presence of new onset or refractory spasms; 2) the kind of aetiology associated with IS; 3) psychomotor development before spasm onset; 4) the presence of systemic diseases such as heart, kidney and metabolic disorders.

The choice of treatment is different if we are in presence of resistant spasms that previously have been treated with steroids or vigabatrin; in such cases, one of the old or new antiepileptic drugs or even non pharmacological treatments should be tried (Shields, 2002). Secondly, a specific aetiology such as tuberous sclerosis or focal cortical dysplasia could indicate vigabatrin as the first choice drug. Furthermore, the presence of a marked psychomotor delay and/or a significant systemic disease could suggest giving up treatments such as ACTH, potentially associated with life-threatening adverse side effects. However, most of these approaches are rather empirical.

Table I shows the different treatment options available for infantile spasms. ACTH/corticosteroids and vigabatrin are considered the mainstay. Only anecdotal evidence is available for some of the old and new antiepileptic drugs which are discussed in this report.

Immunoglobulins, pyridoxine and TRH may control spasms in some patients. Ketogenic diet has also been tried.

As to the main trials available to date on this subject, randomised controlled trials are listed in *Table II*. In the first two studies ACTH has been compared with prednisone, while in the other two studies high dose ACTH was compared with low-dose ACTH. An additional five studies compared vigabatrin with hydrocortisone or with prednisolone/ACTH, or *versus* placebo. In an additional trial a low-dose and a high-dose of vigabatrin were compared. Three other studies evaluated ACTH *versus* nitrazepam, valproate *versus* placebo, and methysergide *versus* alpha-metilparathyrosine, respectively.

A review of the currently available treatments for infantile spasms as well as a critical exposure of the main literature data will be carried on in the following paragraphs. A proposal for a therapeutic scheme for the treatment of infantile spasms based on the data reviewed is presented at the end of this chapter.

ACTH/corticosteroids

The therapeutic effect of ACTH against seizures was first reported by Klein and Livingstone (1950), who observed a beneficial effect of ACTH treatment in four of six children ranging in age from 4.5 to 16 years who were suffering from a variety of seizure types refractory to standard medical therapy. Sorel and Dusaucy-Baulaye (1958) first reported the use of ACTH in seven children with infantile spasms who also presented developmental regression at the onset of spasms. ACTH led to spasm cessation, EEG and psychomotor normalization. Since then there have been a multitude of articles on ACTH and corticosteroid treatment of infantile spasms. Most are retrospective reports, few are prospective open trials, and only five are comparative, controlled trials. In addition, a wide range of treatment schedules is on record.

Table I. Drug options for the treatment of infantile spasms

• ACTH, steroids	• Nitrazepam, clonazepam
• Vigabatrin	• Zonisamide
• Valproate	• Levetiracetam
• Topiramate	• Sulthiame
• Lamotrigine	• Immunoglobulins,
• Felbamate	• Pyridoxine
• Liposteroids	• TRH
	• Ketogenic diet

Table II. RCT trials on infantile spasms

Hrachovy 1983	ACTH/Prednisone
Baram 1996	ACTH/Prednisone
Hrachowy 1994	ACTH high dose/ACTH low dose
Yanagaki 1999	ACTH high dose/ACTH low dose
Chiron 1997	Vigabatrin/Hydrocortisone
Vigevano 1997	Vigabatrin/Hydrocortisone
Appleton 1999	Vigabatrin/Placebo
Elterman 2001	Low dose VGB/High dose VGB
Lux 2004	Vigabatrin/prednisone or ACTH
Dyken 1985	Valproate/Placebo
Hrachowy 1989	Methysergide/Alpha-metilparathyrosine
Dreifuss 1986	ACTH/Nitrazepam
Debus 2004	Sulthiame/placebo

Relative to ACTH, seven randomised controlled studies are currently available. None was placebo controlled and two were cross over studies using prednisone (Hrachowy et al., 1983) or vigabatrin (Vigevano et al., 1997). Two additional studies compared high-dose versus low-dose ACTH (Hrachovy et al., 1994; Yanagaki et al., 1999). Children ranged in age from one to 24 months and all trials used video-EEG monitoring to document a treatment response. Two studies used synthetic ACTH (Vigevano et al., 1997; Yanagaki et al., 1999). ACTH dosage varied from 0.2 IU/kg up to 150 IU/m^2/day and duration of treatment at the highest dose ranged from 7 to 40 days with total treatment time varying from three to 12 weeks. Cessation of spasms was reported in 54% to 87% of patients, with a time from initiation of treatment to cessation of spasms ranging from 7 to 12 days. In almost all randomised controlled trials, a greater percentage of cryptogenic patients responded to ACTH.

ACTH was first compared with prednisone in a double-blind placebo-controlled, crossover study (Hrachovy et al., 1983), in which twenty-four patients with infantile spasms were randomised to ACTH (20-30 IU/day) or prednisone (2 mg/kg/day). Effectiveness of both these treatment options was almost overlapping. Most patients responded within two weeks of initiation of therapy. Few patients had a relapse and four responded rapidly to a second course of therapy. In a second RCT trial (Baram et al., 1996), high-dose corticotropin (ACTH) (150 IU/m^2/day) was compared with prednisone (2 mg/kg/day) given for two weeks in 29 infants with mostly infantile spasms, with a mean age of 6 months. ACTH controlled 86% patients, and prednisone 28.5%. The authors concluded that a 2-week course of high-dose ACTH is superior to 2-weeks of prednisone.

In two other prospective trials (Hrachovy et al., 1994; Yanagaki et al., 1999), high-dose and low-dose ACTH therapy were compared, though in the trial from Hrachovy et al. much higher doses were tested (150 IU/m^2/day vs 20-30 IU/kg/day, and 0.2 IU/kg vs 1 IU/m²/day, respectively). Both these trials showed no major difference in the effectiveness of these two regimens with reference to spasm cessation and improvement of hypsarrhythmic EEG pattern. Adverse side effects were almost overlapping both in the high and low-dose groups, though some of them were significantly milder in the latter group. Relapse rate was 15-35%.

In another RCT trial, ACTH was compared with vigabatrin (see also the section about vigabatrin) as first-line treatment for IS (Vigevano et al., 1997). Forty-two children aged 2-9 months, were randomised to receive vigabatrin (100-150 mg/kg/day) or ACTH (10 IU/day). Overall, spasm control was achieved in 78% patients with ACTH, and in 48% with VGB. ACTH resulted as more effective than VGB in spasms due to perinatal hypoxic-ischemic brain injury, while VGB better controlled spasms due to cerebral malformations and tuberous sclerosis. Three months after initiating treatment, the relapse rate was higher in children treated with ACTH.

A recent multicentre, randomised controlled trial compared vigabatrin to prednisone or to tetracosactide for infantile spasms (Lux et al., 2004). The primary outcome was cessation of spasms on days 13 and 14. Dosages ranged from 100 to 150 mg/kg/day for vigabatrin, oral prednisolone 40 mg/day, and tetracosactide depot 0.5 (40 IU) to 0.75 (60 IU). On days 13 and 14 proportions with no spasms were: 73% of the 55 infants assigned hormonal treatments (prednisolone 70% and tetracosactide 76%, respectively), and 54% of the 52 infants assigned vigabatrin. This study stated that cessation of spasms is more likely in infants given hormonal treatment than those given vigabatrin.

These results were completely reversed by the 12-14 month follow-up study of these infants (Lux et a., 2005). At 12-14 months of age, absence of spasms was similar in each treatment group (75% hormone vs 76% vigabatrin). Based on these results, hormone treatment initially controls spasms better than vigabatrin but in the long-run, no major difference between the two types of treatment can be evidenced. Furthermore, better initial control of spasms by hormone treatment occurred in those with no identified underlying aetiology, which may lead to improved developmental outcome.

There were four prospective open label studies (Hrachovy et al., 1980; Lombroso, 1983; Snead et al., 1989; Kusse et al., 1993). Hrachovy et al. reported that all five children in their series responded to low-dose ACTH, whereas Snead et al. (1989) reported a 93% response rate in 15 children treated with high-dose therapy. Relapse rates were 20% and 36%, respectively. Lombroso (1983) compared the efficacy of synthetic ACTH to oral corticosteroids and benzodiazepines. This study was stratified for symptomatic/cryptogenic aetiology. In the 69 symptomatic patients treated with ACTH, 39% had cessation of spasms and EEG normalised in 32% of patients. Use of ACTH fragments (Kusse et al., 1993) resulted in cessation of spasms in 33% of cases.

The majority of studies on the use of ACTH are retrospective. They reported a response rate for the cessation of spasms ranging from 42% to 100% and a resolution of hypsarrhythmia from 23% to 97%. Relapse rate however ranged from 12% to 47%.

In a multi-institutional study (Ito et al., 2002), the initial effects, adverse effects, and long-term outcome in 138 Japanese children treated for the first time with low-dose synthetic ACTH therapy, have been reported. The daily dosage of synthetic ACTH

(Cotrosyn -Z; hydroxide suspension of tetracosactide acetate) ranged from 0.005 to 0.032 mg/kg body weight (0.2 to 1.26 IU/kg/day). ACTH was injected daily for one to 5 weeks, then stopped or the frequency of injections was reduced over a maximum of 8 weeks. The total dosage of synthetic ACTH ranged from 0.1 to 0.87 mg/kg (4 to 34.8 IU/kg). The mean age of the patients in this study was about 8 months. At the end of ACTH therapy, 106 of 138 (76%) patients showed total cessation of spasms, and 23 (17%) had a decrease of seizure frequency by 50%. The initial effect on EEG was rated as excellent in 53 of 138 (38%) patients, and good in 76 (55%) of patients. Overall response was somewhat better in cryptogenic cases (96%) than symptomatic (73%). At the time of follow-up (more than 2 years), 52% of patients were seizure-free, whereas 48% of patients had seizure persistence. In this study, the factors that correlated with a good initial effect of ACTH included cryptogenic aetiology, age at onset over three months, and a short-term lag. The outcome of WS depended mostly on the aetiology. Thus these results suggest that the dosage of synthetic ACTH used for such patients can be reduced as much as possible to avoid serious side effects.

The same results with extremely low dose ACTH were reported by Oguni et al. (2006). The authors treated 31 children with West syndrome (9 cryptogenic, 22 symptomatic) using synthetic ACTH-Z at a dose of 0.005 mg/kg (= 0.2 IU)/kg/day, injected once every morning for at least two weeks, up to a maximum of 3 weeks. This treatment protocol led to seizure control of both spasms and hypsarrhythmia in 55% of patients, while an additional dosage of 0.025 mg (= 1 IU)/kg/day for the next two weeks allowed seizure control in other two patients. Regarding the long-term effects, 13 patients (48%) with excellent short-term results and a longer than 1-year follow-up remained seizure-free. These authors state that the dose expected to be effective in controlling infantile spasms may be smaller than the dose they previously used. Other Japanese studies (Kondo et al., 2005) reported excitingly good results in controlling IS obtained with ACTH-Z doses ranging between 0.2 to 0.4 IU/kg/day (that means that an 8-month infant weighing about 9 kg should receive 1.6-3.2 IU of ACTH/day for 2-4 weeks).

ACTH has been reported to be effective also for epileptic spasms without hypsarrhytmia (Oguni et al., 2005). Thirty patients were treated with ACTH therapy, and excellent response was obtained in 17 (63%) patients, as a short-term effect. Unfortunately, only about 29% of patients continued to be seizure-free at 21-year follow-up. Considering these results, ACTH is worth trying for patients with spasms and no features of WS, but long-term effect appears uncertain because of recurrence of various types of seizures.

The relapse rate was between 15% and 33% in all these studies. Previous trials reported a relapse rate from 33% (Harris, 1964) to 56% (Jeavons et al., 1973), following the first course of steroid treatment. Relapse usually occurs within 2 months following treatment cessation. A second steroid course may give a response in 74% of cases (Riikonen, 1984). Complete recovery of mental function was found in 6% (Ito et al., 2002) to 58% (Lerman and Kivity, 1982) of patients. Mental outcome seems to greatly depend on aetiology and improvement is more likely in cryptogenic cases (31% by Lombroso et al., 1983; to 56% by Lerman and Kivity, 1982).

Corticosteroids-ganoxolone

In two randomised controlled trials (Hrachovy et al., 1983; Baram et al., 1996), in two prospective trials (Hrachovy et al., 1979; Lombroso, 1983) and in one retrospective trial (Snead et al., 1983), 2 mg/kg/day prednisone for 1-2 months achieved a response rate of 29-42%. Spasm control was better in cryptogenic cases. EEG normalised in about 35-40% of cases. Though the response rate using oral prednisone was not different from that expected with no treatment, based on a limited natural history (Mackay et al., 2004), it is difficult to believe that spasm control achieved within two weeks might have been by pure chance. As compared with ACTH, oral corticosteroids were less effective than high-dose ACTH. In another trial (Hrachovy et al., 1983), prednisone also resulted less effective in normalizing the EEG. Among steroids, there are neurosteroids that are synthetised entirely from cholesterol in the peripheral or central nervous system. They are endogenous steroids that act directly on neuronal ion channels to modify brain excitability. Neuroactive steroids therefore have a wide spectrum of potential therapeutic applications, including treatment of epilepsy. Deoxycorticosterone is their precursor, that is greatly increased by ACTH therapy. Member of a novel class of neuroactive steroids is ganaxolone, which allosterically modulates the gamma aminobutyric acid-A (GABAa) receptor complex in the brain via a unique recognition site (Lee et al., 1995). Ganaxolone was evaluated in a multicentre, open-label, add-on trial (Kerrigan et al., 2000), on 20 children, aged 7 months to 7 years, with refractory infantile spasms, whose frequency was reduced by at least 50% in 33% of them. Ganaxolone was well tolerated. Other compounds of this class are under evaluation for refractory epilepsy.

Adverse effects

The adverse side effects of ACTH and oral corticosteroids are well known. Hypertension is reported in up to 37% of patients, irritability in 37% to 100%, infection in 14%, and reversible brain shrinking in 62% of patients. Hypertension and brain shrinkage are more common with high-doses and may be life threatening in some cases.

Long-term outcome

Prospective and retrospective studies (Matsumoto et al., 1981; Riikonen et al., 1982; Hrachovy et al., 1983; Glaze et al., 1988) indicate that cryptogenic spasms have a better long-term outcome, and that a short treatment lag and a better long-term response to ACTH are associated with a better long-term prognosis. Additional factors of good prognosis include normal development prior to the onset of spasms, no neurological deficits, absence of other seizure types and of other EEG abnormalities after the disappearance of hypsarrhythmia.

In a recent study by Kivity et al. (2004), early treatment (within one month from onset) of cryptogenic spasms with a high dose ACTH protocol (tetracosactide depot, 1 mg IM every 48 hours for two months) is associated with favorable long-term cognitive outcome. In patients treated after 1 to 6.5 months, a normal outcome was observed in only 40% of patients. This trial concluded that early treatment is mandatory in order to obtain a favorable outcome.

Vigabatrin

Vigabatrin is an irreversible inhibitor of gaba-transaminase that has proven effective for the treatment of infantile spasms due to different aetiologies and in particular tuberous sclerosis (Chiron 1997). In one of the four randomised controlled trials in which VGB was used, Appleton et al. (1999) supported the results of previously published open and prospective trials (Vles et al., 1993; Siemes et al., 1998). In this study, forty children with newly diagnosed infantile spasms received either VGB or placebo for 5 days in a double-blind, placebo-controlled, parallel-group study, after which all the infants continuing the study were treated openly with VGB for a minimum of 24 weeks. Compared with baseline, at the end of the double-blind phase, patients on VGB had a 78% reduction in spasms compared to 26% in the plaxebo group, seven (35%) patients treated with VGB were spasm-free and five (25%) had resolution of hypsarrhythmia. Relapse was seen in four (20%) of vigabatrin-treated patients. Of note, is that VGB resulted effective on all aetiologies of IS. In another randomised trial, Chiron et al. (1997) treated for one month 22 infants with tuberous sclerosis of which 11 with vigabatrin (150 mg/kg/day), and 11 with hydrocortisone (HC) (15 mg/kg/day). All vigabatrin treated patients were spasm-free *versus* 5 of the on HC. Further, the infants crossed to vigabatrin for inefficacy of HC, also became totally controlled. On the basis of these results the authors considered VGB to be superior to steroids for the treatment of infantile spasms due to TSC. In another prospective randomised trial, Elterman et al. (2002) found that VGB was more effective at high doses (100-140 mg/kg/day) than at low doses (18-36 mg/kg/day), and confirmed that this drug was particularly effective in IS due to TSC.

In new onset cases, VGB monotherapy is more effective in children starting before the age of 3 months (over 90 per cent) than in those starting later (Aicardi et al., 1996).The rate of total suppression of spasms in newly diagnosed cases depends on aetiology. It reached 90% in tuberous sclerosis, and focal cortical dysplasia, and about 70% in cryptogenic cases with no previous psychomotor delay (Dulac and Tuxhorn, 2005).

In a controlled trial, VGB was compared to steroids (Lux et al., 2004) in patients with infantile spasms due to all other conditions than tuberous sclerosis. In this UK multicenter trial, Lux et al. (2004) found that the cessation of spasms was more likely in infants given hormonal treatments (73%) than those given vigabatrin (54%). Of note, is that hypsarrhythmia resolved in more infants on hormonal treatments than on vigabatrin (81% vs 56%, respectively). Adverse events were equally common with both treatments. Response to treatment was not affected by the underlying cause.

In another controlled trial, Vigevano and Cilio (1997) compared adrenocorticotropin hormone depot injection (10 IU daily thought to be equivalent to 10 IU tetracosactide) with vigabatrin (100-150 mg/kg/day). If we exclude a few infants with tuberous sclerosis, a better response to hormonal treatment (13 out of 18 infants) than to VGB (8 of 20) was found, thus supporting the data from Lux et al. (2004). Vigevano and Cilio reported a trend towards more adverse events with hormonal treatments (37% vs 13% with VGB). Furthermore, they found a higher rate of relapses with steroids.

If the last two studies prove a better initial control of spasms by hormone treatment than vigabatrin, a 12 month follow-up reverses this result, confirming that absence of spasms is similar in each treatment group (74% and 76%, respectively) (Lux et al., 2005).

Villeneuve et al. (1998) and Granstrom et al. (1999) reported on a particular group of patients with psychomotor delay prior to the first spasms and no MRI abnormalities, who required the combination of both VGB and steroids to get under control, and a duration of treatment of more than 3 months in order to prevent relapses.

Side effects due to VGB are overall milder than steroids, although they may be as frequent. They mainly consist of irritability, agitation, weight gain and insomnia. Major concerns come from the risk of visual field defect (Wild et al., 1999; Vanhatolo et al., 1999; Iannetti et al., 2000), which is irreversible. To date, a single report of reduced visual function in children with infantile spasms and a history of vigabatrin use has been published (Hammoudi et al., 2005). Contrast sensitivity and visual acuity were reduced in vigabatrin-treated children with infantile spasms, compared with vigabatrin-treated children with other seizure disorders and healthy control subjects. But these authors conclude that the visual defect is probably associated with infantile spasms rather than vigabatrin. In addition, cumulative doses have been shown to play a potential role (Vanhatolo et al., 2002). Consequently, a proposal of reducing the duration of VGB treatment has been carried out (Nabbout et al., 2001; Capovilla et al., 2004). VGB is not commercially available in the United States.

■ Valproic acid

Valproic acid has been initially tried in small series for the treatment of infantile spasms, at daily doses ranging from 20 to 60 mg/kg, and leading to spasm cessation in up to 40% of patients (Pavone et al., 1981). The drug was overall well tolerated and the authors considered it to be a first-line treatment option and suggested the use of hormonal treatment only in unresponsive patients. Dyken et al. (1985) tried VPA in patients who failed to respond to adenocorticotropin (ACTH) or corticosteroid therapy and found to be beneficial.

Siemes et al. (1988) reported on 22 children with mostly symptomatic infantile spasms, who were given 40-100 mg/kg/day valproic acid, achieving a seizure control in about 50%. Such results were obtained within 1 month, with VPA blood levels between 46 and 77 microgr/dl. In six children there were severe relapses during the first 7 months of therapy. Hypotonia and somnolence were the most frequent adverse side effects. Similar results were achieved by Prats et al. (1991) in 42 patients with infantile spasms who were given higher doses of valproic acid (100-300 mg/kg/day). In 75% of patients, control of the hypsarrhythmic pattern was reached after 2 weeks, but with significant adverse events, including trombocytopenia, severe vomiting and mild somnolence. In the same year, Ito et al. (1991) treated 20 children with infantile spasms with high-dose Vit. B6 or with valproic acid or a combination of both. Vit. B6 combined with valproic acid was found more effective than Vit. B6 alone, with reference to spasm frequency and EEG abnormalities. In addition, ACTH had an excellent effect on seizures in 86% of the patients who did not respond well to vitamin B6, valproic acid or both.

Anecdotical cases have been reported in which valproate was associated with dose-related and idiosyncratic hepatotoxicity (Fenichel and Grenne,1985; Go et al., 2002). The dose-related adverse event may cause alterations in liver function, but is not associated with death. Conversely, idiosyncratic hepatotoxicity is rare, usually irreversible, and not predictable on the basis of laboratory monitoring. Valproate cannot be used in cases suspected to suffer from a urea cycle or a fatty acid oxydation disorders.

■ Topiramate

Topiramate was first tried for the therapy of refractory infantile spasms in a pilot study (Glauser et al., 1998) in which 11 infants, most of them symptomatic, were given an initial dose of 25 mg TPM per day in addition to their current therapy. Because of the necessity of controlling the symptoms as quickly as possible, dosage was increased by 25 mg every 2-3 days until spasms were controlled, the maximal tolerated dose was reached, or the maximal dose of 24 mg/kg/day was achieved. Nine infants with five of them becoming seizure free (45%) achieved a spasm reduction of > 50%. The remissions occurred on days 6 and 11 in two children, at TPM doses ranging from 6.7 to 8.8 mg/kg/day, and in three additional children on days 32, 36, and 90 after their first TPM dose, at doses ranging from 19.2 to 29.9 mg/kg/day. The most reported adverse events during TPM treatment were irritability and sleep disturbance, that in a few cases required a temporary dose reduction.

The mean dose of TPM during stabilization was 15.0 ± 5.7 mg/kg/day. Rapid TPM dosing appeared to be well tolerated in these very young children.

Four out of seven patients with refractory infantile spasms became seizure free in a retrospective study (Thijs et al., 2001), in which TPM was given at the daily doses of 2-24 mg/kg body weight. Less encouraging were more recent data from Mikaeloff et al. (2003). Of 14 patients with infantile spasms, some responded (43%), but some worsened (29%) with topiramate. No patients became seizure free. The mean daily dose of TPM was 4.5 mg/kg far below that of 15.0 ± 5.7 mg/kg administered by Glauser et al. (1998). Nevertheless, Mikaeloff et al. state that there was no clear benefit when increasing the dose. It has been suggested that better results with TPM may be achieved in combination with vigabatrin (Buoni et al., 2004).

■ Lamotrigine

Reports on lamotrigine (LTG) use for patients with IS are rare. Veggiotti et al., (1994) described 30 children with refractory infantile spasms, to whom LTG was administered as adjunctive treatment. Sixteen of the 30 children became seizure free and the remaining showed > 50% decrease in spasm frequency. LTG was overall well tolerated.

Another report described the use of LTG therapy in 13 infants, seven of whom had IS (Mikati et al., 2002). The mean age of these patients was 3.66 months at the time of initiation of LTG, and 11 of them were less than 2 months old, which is an unusual age for infantile spasm onset. The dosage and titration of LTG were based on whether the child was receiving concomitant P450 enzyme-inducing drugs, with a final dosage of 10-20 mg/kg/day for patients on enzyme-inducers and

5-10 mg/kg/day for those on non inducers. Spasm frequency significantly decreased 8.71 +/− 2.15 to 3.61 +/− 2.76 per day (p = 0.028), and five of seven IS had a 75-100% decrease in spasm frequency.

Cianchetti et al., (2002) described three patients with IS who were unresponsive to VGB and ACTH, but responded rapidly to low doses LTG, achieving seizure freedom.

■ Felbamate

Felbamate has been reported to be useful in infantile spasms. One small open-label study (Hosain et al., 1997) studied felbamate as add-on therapy in 11 children aged 6 to 45 months who had treatment-resistant infantile spasms. Felbamate was initiated at 15 mg/kg/d and titrated to 45 mg/kg/d by weeks 3 to 6. Two patients required doses up to 60 and 75 mg/kg/d.

In patients who were receiving valproate at the onset of the study, the dose was decreased by 25% on felbamate initiation. Valproate then was tapered and discontinued in all patients. The median follow-up for all patients was 22 weeks. The median decrease in seizure frequency, as measured by seizure counts from baseline and treatment video EEG segments, was 72%. The median decrease in electrodecremental events was 73%. A reduction in clinical spasms was noted in seven patients overall ($P < .05$), as was a decrease in electrodecremental events.

Caregiver data revealed improvement in the frequency of infantile spasms in 10 patients ($P < .05$). Greater clinical improvement was observed in patients who had an earlier onset of seizures ($P = .02$). Felbamate was generally well tolerated. Dose-related adverse effects included weight loss in one patient and increased vomiting in a child with gastroesophageal reflux. Both effects resolved with dose reduction. Several case reports of children aged 5 to 24 months with refractory infantile spasms describe improvement in or complete control of seizures after 2 to 4 days of therapy with 15 to 45 mg/kg/d of felbamate; all the children were reported to be more alert (Hurst and Rolan, 1995). Unfortunately, aplastic anemia has an incidence of approximately 127 cases per million patients on felbamate (~1:8000). Thirty-one cases of aplastic anemia were reported to the US Food and Drug Administration between January 1994 and January 1995, of which 7 resulted in death. Aside from these two potentially fatal reactions, the most commonly reported adverse events during clinical trials in children receiving felbamate were anorexia, somnolence, insomnia, vomiting, weight loss, nausea, and gait abnormalities. The risk of such potentially life-threatening events consistently limit the use of this drug.

■ Liposteroid

Liposteroid is dexamethasone palmitate incorporated into liposomes and was developed as an anti-inflammatory drug for targeting therapy mainly for rheumatoid arthritis. Yamamoto et al. (1998) first used liposteroid for the treatment of West syndrome and compared it with adrenocorticotropic hormone (ACTH) therapy. Five infants aged 4 to 11 months with symptomatic infantile spasms received a single intravenous injection of liposteroid (0.25 mg/kg; total dosage 1.75 mg/kg), seven times during a three month period. An additional five symptomatic patients, aged 6-10 months, were administered ACTH (0.025 mg/kg/day) for 6 weeks. Nodding spasms and hypsarrhythmia on EEG disappeared within four doses in all patients treated with liposteroid therapy; however, 3 out of 5 patients developed partial seizures and focal spikes on EEG two months after the end of liposteroid therapy. In the ACTH therapy group, spasms and EEG abnormalities disappeared in all patients but partial seizures recurred in 3 children as well. Liposteroid therapy was overall well tolerated thus suggesting liposteroid to be a suitable therapy for infantile spasms. Encouraging results were also obtained by Yoshikawa et al. (2000) in 3 children with epileptic encephalopaties, while Shimono et al.(2003) achieved only transient and partial improvement in 6 patients with refractory infantile spasms.

■ Nitrazepam and other benzodiazepines

Certain 1,4-benzodiazepines have shown to be effective against infantile spasms. Among these, nitrazepam has been studied in clinical trials (Volzke et al., 1967; Dreifuss et al., 1986; Chamberlain, 1996). Dreifuss et al. enrolled 52 patients with IS in a four-week randomised multicenter controlled study comparing nitrazepam and corticotropin. All patients were less than 2 years of age. Both treatment resulted in statistically significant reduction in spasm frequency from that at baseline, but with no significant differences among treatments. The number of patients who experienced adverse side effects were similar in the two treatment groups, but those encountered among the patients treated with corticotropin were qualitatively more severe. Chamberlain et al., (1996) treated 20 children aged 4 to 28 months, affected by medically refractory infantile spasms or the Lennox-Gastaut syndrome, in an open label study. Daily dosage of nitrazepam ranged from 0.5 to 3.5 mg/kg, with a median dosage of 1.5 mg/kg, divided into two doses per day. A 25% response rate was obtained throughout the study and serious side effects were seen, including pooling of oral secretions and sedation. Furthermore, clonazepam (Vassella et al., 1973) and clobazam (Silva et al., 2006) have been shown to be effective against infantile spasms, as well. However, their usefulness is limited by deleterious side effects such drowsiness, generalised hypotonia and increased bronchial secretions. Additionally, they may be somewhat effective on seizure frequency, but they poorly modify the EEG hypsarrhythmic pattern.

■ Zonisamide

Among the new antiepileptic drugs on the market, zonisamide has been tried as add-on drug in the treatment of infantile spasms. Marketed in Japan in 1989 and available in the USA since 2000, ZNS has been reported by many authors as effective in decreasing spasm frequency and severity in 20-30% of cases (Yanay et al., 1999; Suzuki et al., 1997, 2002), with a better response in cryptogenic (29% to 100%) than in symptomatic spasms (15% to 53%). However, treatment regimen, previous and concomitant medications and the definition of response were variable in these open studies and the results obtained difficult to evaluate.

Recently, Lotze et al., (2004) evaluated ZNS for the treatment of symptomatic infantile spasms in 23 patients, aged 2 to 47 months (range 12 months), with a mean age at clinical spasm onset of 9 months (2-42 months). Zonisamide was started at the mean daily dosage of 6.2 mg/kg (range 1-11 mg), with a maximum dosage of 18 mg/kg (range 8-32 mg). Zonisamide was initiated as primary therapy in 10 patients (43%). Complete spasm control (*i.e.* complete spasm cessation and clearing of hypsarrhythmia) was achieved within 14-35 days in six patients (26%) of whom five are currently achieving ZNS as monotherapy. Adverse effects were anorexia in 5 patients (21%) and weight loss in one. Cryptogenic spasm patients showed a better response rate than those with symptomatic spasms. A drawback of this treatment is the considerable time lag to achieve seizure freedom.

■ Levetiracetam

To date, levetiracetam (LEV) has been tried for the treatment of infantile spasms in a few sporadic cases. Lawlor and Devlin (2005) reported an 11-month-old infant with a 5-month history of seizures and a 3-month history of infantile spasms. Spasms were resistant to treatment with clobazam. Following the introduction of LEV, there was clinical cessation of seizures with resolution of seizure activity on the EEG. One further study from Lagae et al. (2003), reported a good efficacy of LEV in one patient with infantile spasms.

■ Sulthiame

Sulthiame (STM), a sulphonamide derivative and carboanhydrase inhibitor, is commonly used in some countries for the treatment of idiopathic focal epilepsies (Ben-Zeev et al., 2004), and has been recently tried against infantile spasms by Debus et al.(2004) in a prospective, randomised placebo-controlled study. Thirty-seven infants with newly diagnosed WS, aged between 3.5 and 15 months, received baseline therapy with pyridoxine. The children were randomised to STM (n = 20) or placebo (n = 17) starting at day 4 at a moderate dose of 5 mg/kg body weight. In absence of complete cessation of spasms and resolution of hypsarrhythmia, the dose was doubled at day 7. Six out of 20 children (30%) responded to STM, but three patients with tuberous sclerosis had no response. This author states that STM may be effective in IS.

■ Immunoglubulins

Immunological disturbances were found to be more prominent in children with infantile spasms, consisting mainly in cell-mediated deficiencies and low levels of immunoglubulins in some patients (Mantelli et al., 1984; Mota et al., 1984). In addition Siemes et al., (1984) found in 50 children with both symptomatic and cryptogenic infantile spasms, an increased permeability of the blood CSF barrier, especially for albumin. Changes were most marked in the symptomatic group, and slight in the cryptogenic group. All patients treated with ACTH or dexametasone showed the reappearance of normal cerebrovascular permeability for protein. Based on these data, high-dose non-treated immunoglobulin therapy was administered intravenously to six children with cryptogenic infantile spasms and to five patients with symptomatic spasms (Ariizumi et al., 1987). Immunoglubulins were given at 100-200 mg/kg of body weight at intervals of 2 or 3 weeks. All patients with cryptogenic spasms showed complete seizure remission; conversely, only 1 out of 5 symptomatic patients became seizure-free. These Authors concluded that high doses of immunogloblulins may be useful for early treatment of cryptogenic infantile spasms. A few years later, Echenne et al. (1991) treated 23 infants with infantile spasms with intravenous gammaglobulins at high doses. None of the patients had recently undergone corticosteroid therapy. Fifteen out of 23 patients showed no effect, while transitory clinical and/or EEG improvement was noted in three. Only 5 patients developed complete normalization, of whom 4 had severe brain lesions. The whole results of this trial was defined as disappointing. However, the spectacular clinical and electroencephalographic improvement in some cases may suggest that I.V. gammaglobulins be used as auxiliary treatment in infantile spasms. Finally, no correlations were found between therapeutical results and immunological abnormalities.

A few cases in whom spasm reduction averaged 50%-70% have been reported in recent years (Van Engelen et al., 1994; Bingel et al., 2003).

■ Pyridoxine

Pryridoxine and its active metabolite pyridoxal-phosphate have been given at high doses, alone or in combination with ACTH or sulthiame, for the treatment of infantile spasms. Ohtsuka et al. (1987) first found effective high doses of pyridoxal phosphate (PAL-P) in 15 (12.7%) of 118 infants with West syndrome. Spasms were completely suppressed in 12 cases by PAL-P alone, and in other 3 children in whom it had been given as add-on to therapy. At follow-up, 12 cases have continued to be free from seizures, while two cases relapsed in the Lennox-Gastaut syndrome, and one died. The hypsarrhythmic EEG disappeared by PAL-P in all 15 effective cases. The efficacious daily doses of PAL-P were 30 to 400 mg. Notably, PAL-P was effective even in presence of obvious organic lesions such as tuberous sclerosis, poroencephaly, holoprosencephaly, postmeningitis, besides 5 idiopathic cases. PAL-P was significantly more effective in idiopathic cases. These Authors suggest a treatment with a high-dose PAL-P should be tried in all cases of the West syndrome at first. In another trial (Pietz et al., 1993), high-dose vitamin B6 (Pyridoxine-HCL, 300 mg/kg/day, orally) was introduced as the initial treatment of recently manifested spasms in 17 children of whom 13 were symptomatic and 4 cryptogenic cases. Five out of 17 (3 cryptogenic and 2 symptomatic) were classified as responders. In all cases the response occurred within the first 2 weeks of treatment. In 2 children other seizures manifested, but no infantile spasms relapsed. No serious adverse reactions were noted, side effects being mainly gastrointestinal symptoms, which disappeared after reduction of the daily dose. High dose pyridoxal-phosphate (40-50 m/kg/day) has been combined with low-dose ACTH (0.01/mg/day) leading to spasm control by 90% in two small series including a total of 43 patients. Response was achieved within 1 month, and spasms recurred in 29% of patients (Seki et al., 1990; Takuma, et al., 1998). Pyridoxal-phospate was found to be better than pyridoxine for controlling idiopathic intractable epilepsy, including infantile spasms (Wang et al., 2005). Recently, 12 children with infantile spasms pretreated with pyridoxine (150-300 mg/kg/day) for a few days showed spasm control in 58% of cases after sulthiame (10 mg/kg/day) was added to previous therapy. None of the patients responded to pyridoxine alone (Debus et al., 2004).

■ Thyrotropin-releasing hormone (TRH)

Thyrotropin-releasing hormone and selected analogs have been reported to exert antiepileptic effects in several animal models, including electroconvulsive shock and kindling.

In 1981, Inanaga et al. reported on the efficacy of a TRH analog in the treatment of degenerative myoclonus epilepsy and other forms of refractory epilepsy. Following this report, Matsuishi et al. (1983) studied the efficacy and safety of TRH treatment in 10 resistant epileptic children aged between 6 months and 11 years, including 7 with Lennox syndrome and 2 with West syndrome. TRH was administered at the daily dose of 0.02-0.05 mg/kg, initially, and then was increased to 0.05 mg/kg. A less than 50% decrease in spasm frequency was reported in the two IS patients. Activation of psychomotor activity was also noted. A few years later, Matsumoto et al. (1987) investigated the clinical and side effects of TRH in 31 out of 64 patients with severe childhood epilepsy. Seven out of 13 infants with infantile spasms, achieved complete seizure control, and a marked improvement of EEGs was observed in 8 of 13 of them. TRH was well tolerated, and only 16% of patients had transient reduction of urine volume.

Among the various factors possibly influencing responsiveness to TRH therapy, serum prolactin level was found to significantly correlate (the higher the PRL, the greater the response rate) in a study regarding 16 children by Matsumoto et al. (1989). In another trial (Takeuchi et al. 1995), no significant differences in monoamine metabolites before and after TRH administration were found, even though the same author found increased concentrations of kynurenine (an antagonist of the NMDA receptor complex) in cerebrospinal fluid of 14 TRH-treated patients. The results of this study may explain at least one of the mechanisms of the effectiveness of TRH therapy in intractable epilepsy. Although TRH has not yet widely studied as a treatment of refractory epilepsy outside Japan, it might be considered as a possible new strategy for treating West and Lennox syndromes prior to ACTH, especially for the patient with infection, immunosuppression, or severe organic lesions in the brain (Takeuchi et al., 2001).

■ Ketogenic diet

Ketogenic diet is part of the treatment options for patients with intractable or refractory epilepsy, other than antiepileptic drugs, including surgery and vagal nerve stimulation. It is a high-fat, adequate protein, low carbohydrate diet developed in 1920s. In recent years, ketogenic diet has been revisited mainly in European countries and a number of research publications and media interest have renewed debate on its merits. Overall, ketogenic diet resulted more effective against generalised crypto-symptomatic epilepsy syndromes including infantile spasms. Freeman et al. (1998) first reported KD to be effective in 39% of children with infantile spasms, leading to > 90% seizure reduction. On the basis of this information, Kossoff et al., (2002) expanded their investigation to include other cases of infantile spasms. During a 4-year period, 23 children with infantile spasms, aged 5 months to 2 years, were started on the ketogenic diet; 9 (39%) had symptomatic IS (2 TSC, 2 mitocondrial disease, 1 Down syndrome, 1 22 translocation, 1 right frontal dysgenesis, 1 dysmielination, and 1 bilateral cortical dysgenesis) and 16 (70%) had hypsarrhythmia. Children had an average prediet exposure to 33 anticonvulsants. Two children had KD as first treatment option. All cases were evaluated retrospectively. At 3, 6, 9 and 12 months, 38%, 39%, 53%, and 46%, respectively, of all patients currently on the diet were > 90% improved (3 were seizure-free at 12 months). Fifty-six per cent remained on the diet at 12 months, 46% of whom were > 90% improved. No child died, and 7 children had diet-related adverse reactions, including nephrolitiasis and gastroesophageal reflux. Notably, 6 of 7 children in whom significant reduction in spasms was reported, were younger than 1 year and had only a few months of KD exposure. This might suggest the presence of a critical period of neurological susceptibility in patients with infantile spasms. The fact that this is a retrospective study, based on parental reports that are undoubtedly less accurate than EEG or video-EEG monitoring, and that it is possible that some of the improvement seen in these patients may have been secondary to spontaneous remission, represents significant drawbacks to this study. In the same period, the efficacy and safety of the ketogenic diet was evaluated by Nordli et al. (2001) in a study in which 12 of 17 infants (70%) with infantile spasms had a > 50% improvement on the ketogenic diet. Of note, patients with infantile spasms responded more favorably to the diet than did patients with other specific seizure types. There were no reports of increased seizure frequency on the diet. The effectiveness of the diet was independent of the cause of the epilepsy and seizure type, with the exception that children with infantile spasms/myoclonic seizures responded better than other children. Most children maintained strong ketosis, and parents of infants cited improvements in behavior, alertness and function. Six of the 32 children (18.8%) developed complications possibly related to the diet, including severe vomiting, gastrointestinal bleeding, chronic esophagitis and level of triglicerides over 9,000 mg/dl that resolved after switching to the medium-chain tryglicerides diet.

Two years later, a french trial (Francois et al., 2003) reported that the ketogenic diet improved seizure control in 12 of 29 children, most of them with infantile spasms. Compliance to the diet was good and only one child had hypokaliemia. Recently, Rubenstein et al. (2005) confirmed the efficacy of the ketogenic diet as early therapy in 13 patients of a large series of 460 patients treated with KD at the Johns-Hopkins Hospital. Eight of these 13 infants had infantile spasms and 5 had ketogenic diet as first treatment option. Fat to protein and carbohydrate ratios were 4:1 in five patients and 3:1 in eight patients. Younger patients were started on 3:1 ratios. Six of 8 patients (75%) with IS started on dietary therapy within 1 month of diagnosis responded compared with 3 of 5 patients (60%) with other diagnoses. At 12 month fellow-up, 6 had a more than 90% seizure reduction. In conclusion, even though the ketogenic diet certainly remains harder to initiate and maintain its use is of interest mainly in children with resistant infantile spasms.

Conclusions

Evidence exists for a major clinical efficacy against infantile spasms using ACTH, corticosteroids and vigabatrin. *Table III* (from Shields, 2002, modified) clearly summarizes the relative efficacy of the different treatment options. In synthesis, ACTH seems to be the most effective drug, even though corticosteroids resulted as effective in some trials. Vigabatrin appeared somewhat less efficacious than ACTH (Vigevano *et al.*, 2002), even though the relapse rate was reported to be lesser after ACTH/ steroids treatment. Unfortunately, vigabatrin is consistently limited by the potential tunnel vision side effect reported in about 35 to 40% of patients. Short-term treatment with VGB has been suggested in order to avoid such a risk. Other antiepileptic drugs were variably effective, and their use seems to be limited essentially to refractory spasms. As to the ketogenic diet, more data is needed both for the therapy of new onset and refractory IS to make it a convincing treatment option.

Considering the evidence-based medicine criteria for clinical trials, the American Academy of Neurology and Child Neurology Society (2004) concludes that: "ACTH is *probably* effective for the short-term treatment of epileptic spasms, but there is insufficient evidence to recommend the optimum dosage and duration of treatment. There is insufficient evidence to determine whether oral corticosteroids are effective. Vigabatrin is *possibly* effective for the short-term treatment of epileptic spasms and is *possibly* also effective for children with West syndrome of tuberous sclerosis. There is *insufficient evidence* to recommend any other treatment of epileptic spasms. There is *insufficient evidence* to conclude that successful treatment of epileptic spasms improves the long-term prognosis".

Table III. Efficacy of medical therapies for infantile spasms

Medications used for infantile spasms	Response rate
ACTH, prednisone, or other steroids	~70% with 35-50% relapse
Pyridoxine	11-25%
Vigabatrin	40-90%
Topiramate	45%
Lamotrigine	30%
Valproic acid	15-50%
Zonisamide	25%
Clonazepam	25-50%
Nitrazepam	15-50%
Felbamate	9-75%
Ketogenic diet	40-60%

From Shields, 2002, modified.

The tone of the above conclusion is puzzling as the fact remains that at least some of the available treatments undoubtedly lead to clearcut and often dramatic control of infantile spasms, as demonstrated by our daily clinical practice. As far as the long-term efficacy, it has yet to be fully determined of the successful treatment options. It is also necessary for pharmacological research to offer new therapeutic approaches based, for instance, on the role of the neurotransmission mechanisms, potentially implicated in the genesis of infantile spasms, such as the serotoninergic and dopaminergic neurotransmission. (Aicardi, 2002). The proposal of a therapeutic scheme (*Table IV*; from Shields, 2002, modified) for the treatment of the infantile spasms may then result in more definite treatment conclusions by providing the neuropaediatrician with significant results to review. The aetiology should strongly address the treatment choices, as discussed in the beginning of this review. Symptomatic spasms due for instance to tuberous sclerosis or focal cortical dysplasia may suggest the use of vigabatrin. Cryptogenic/idiopathic cases might preferentially be treated with ACTH/steroids. An initial short-lasting treatment with high-dose pyridoxine is a common protocol, mainly in Japan, followed by a 1-week trial with vigabatrin; in case of inefficacy, ACTH/prednisone is started. If surgical treatment is not indicated, an essay with some of the old and new antiepileptic drugs has to be initiated, including the ketogenic diet and vagal nerve stimulation. Further large studies to evaluate not only spasm cessation but mostly the relationship between the long-term EEG and neuropsychological and mental effects, are always welcome and encouraged.

Table IV. A logical sequence of treatment for West's syndrome

1. Identify the underlying etiology:
   - Symptomatic
     - With specific therapy (i.e. TSC, cortical dysplasia, in born errors of metabolism)
     - Without specific therapy
   - Cryptogenic/idiopathic
2. Initial medical therapies
   - Directed toward specific etiology, if possible
   - Pyridoxine 100-200 mg/dose; short response time)
   - Vigabatrin (short-term treatment)
   - ACTH/prednisone (to be carefully considered in children with symptomatic is and systemic disease i.e. heart/renal failure)
3. If standard approaches fail, assess for the possibility of surgical intervention
4. If the patient is not a surgical candidate or if surgery fails, then consider
   - Valproic acid
   - Topiramate
   - Lamotrigine
   - Levetiracetam
   - Zonisamide
   - Benzodiazepines (clonazopam, nitracepam, clobazam)
   - Ketogenic diet
   - Vagus nerve stimulation

From Shields, 2002.

References

Aicardi J. What we must know to develop better therapies? In *Epilepsy, Infantile Spasms and Developmental Encephalopathy*. Ed. By P. Schwrtzkhroin and J. Rho. Academic Press, 2002: 141-52.

Aicardi J, Mumford JP, Dum C, Wood S. Vigabatrin as initial therapy for infantile spasms: a European retrospective survey. Sabril IS Investigator and Peer Review Groups. *Epilepsia* 1996; 37: 638-42.

Appleton RE, Peters AC, Mumford JP, Shaw DE. Randomised, placebo-controlled study of vigabatrin as first-line treatment of infantile spasms. *Epilepsia* 1999; 40: 1627-33.

Ariizumi M, Baba K, Hibio S *et al*. Immunoglobulin therapy in the West syndrome.

Baram TZ, Mitchell WG, Tournay A, Snead OC, Hanson RA, Horton EJ. High-dose corticotropin (ACTH) *versus* prednisone for infantile spasms: a prospective, randomized, blinded study. *Pediatrics* 1996; 97: 375-9.

Baram TZ. Treatment of infantile spasms: the ideal and the mundane. *Epilepsia* 2003; 44: 993-4.

Ben-Zeev B, Watemberg N, Lerman P, Barash I, Brand N, Lerman-Sagie T. Sulthiame in childhood epilepsy. *Pediatr Int* 2004; 46: 521-4.

Bingel U, Pinter JD, Sotero de Menezes M, Rho JM. Intravenous immunoglobulin as adjunctive therapy for juvenile spasms. *J Child Neurol* 2003; 18: 379-82.

Buoni S, Zannolli R, Strambi M, Fois A. Combined treatment with vigabatrin and topiramate in West syndrome. *J Child Neurol* 2004; 19: 385-6.

Chiron C, Dumas C, Jambaque I, Mumford J, Dulac O. Randomized trial comparing vigabatrin and hydrocortisone in infantile spasms due to tuberous sclerosis. *Epilepsy Res* 1997; 26: 389-95.

Cianchetti C, Pruna D, Coppola G, Pascotto A. Low-dose lamotrigine in West syndrome. *Epilepsy Res* 2002; 51: 199-200.

Debus OM, Kurlemann G; Study group. Sulthiame in the primary therapy of West syndrome: a randomized double-blind placebo-controlled add-on trial on baseline pyridoxine medication. *Epilepsia* 2004; 45: 103-8.

Dreifuss F, Farwell J, Holmes G *et al*. Infantile spasms. Comparative trial of nitrazepam and corticotropin. *Arch Neurol* 1986; 43: 1107-10.

Dulac O, Tuxhorn I. Infantile spasms and West syndrome. In: *Epilepsy: a comprehensive textbook*. Ed. by J Engel Jr. and T.A. Pedley. Lippincott-Raven Publishers, Philadelphia, 1997: 2277-83.

Dyken PR, DuRant RH, Minden DB, King DW. Short term effects of valproate on infantile spasms. *Pediatr Neurol* 1985; 1: 34-7.

Echenne B, Dulac O, Parayre-Chanez MJ *et al*. Treatment of infantile spasms with intravenous gammaglobulins. *Brain Dev* 1991; 13: 313-9.

Elterman RD, Shields WD, Mansfield KA, Nakagawa J; US Infantile Spasms Vigabatrin Study Group. Randomized trial of vigabatrin in patients with infantile spasms. *Neurology* 2001; 57: 1416-21.

Francois LL, Manel V, Rousselle C, David M. Ketogenic regime as anti-epileptic treatment: its use in 29 epileptic children]. *Arch Pediatr* 2003; 10: 300-6.

Freeman JM, Vining EP, Pillas DJ, Pyzik PL, Casey JC, Kelly LM. The efficacy of the ketogenic diet-1998: a prospective evaluation of intervention in 150 children. *Pediatrics* 1998; 102: 1358-63.

Glauser TA, Clark PO, Strawsburg R. A pilot study of topiramate in the treatment of infantile spasms. *Epilepsia* 1998; 39: 1324-8.

Glaze DG, Hrachovy RA, Frost JD Jr, Kellaway P, Zion TE. Prospective study of outcome of infants with infantile spasms treated during controlled studies of ACTH and prednisone. *J Pediatr* 1988; 112: 389-96.

Harris R. Some eeg observations in children with infantile spasms treated with acth. *Arch Dis Child* 1964; 39: 564-70.

Hosain S, Nagarajan L, Carson D, Solomon G, Mast J, Labar D. Felbamate for refractory infantile spasms. *J Child Neurol* 1997; 12: 466-8.

Hrachovy RA, Frost JD Jr, Glaze DG, Rose D. Treatment of infantile spasms with methysergide and alpha-methylparatyrosine. *Epilepsia* 1989; 30: 607-10.

Hrachovy RA, Frost JD Jr, Glaze DG. High-dose, long-duration *versus* low-dose, short-duration corticotropin therapy for infantile spasms. *J Pediatr* 1994; 124: 803-6.

Hrachovy RA, Frost JD Jr, Kellaway P, Zion A controlled study of ACTH therapy in infantile spasms. *Epilepsia* 1980; 21: 631-6.

Hrachovy RA, Frost JD Jr, Kellaway P, Zion T. A controlled study of prednisone therapy in infantile spasms. *Epilepsia* 1979; 20: 403-7.

Hrachovy RA, Frost JD Jr, Kellaway P, Zion TE. Double-blind study of ACTH *vs* prednisone therapy in infantile spasms. *J Pediatr* 1983; 103: 641-5.

Hurst DL, Rolan TD. The use of felbamate to treat infantile spasms. *J Child Neurol* 1995; 10: 134-6.

Inanaga K, Inoue Y. Effect of a thyrotropin releasing hormone analog in a patient with myoclonus epilepsy. *Kurume Med J* 1981; 28: 201-10.

Ito M, Aiba H, Hashimoto K,et Low-dose ACTH therapy for West syndrome: initial effects and long-term outcome. *Neurology*. 2002; 58: 110-4.

Jeavons PM, Bower BD, Dimitrakoudi M. Long-term prognosis of 150 cases of "West syndrome".*Epilepsia* 1973; 14: 153-64.

Kerrigan JF, Shields WD, Nelson TY Ganaxolone for treating intractable infantile spasms: a multicenter, open-label, add-on trial. *Epilepsy Res.* 2000; 42: 133-9.

Kivity S, Lerman P, Ariel R, Danziger Y, Mimouni M, Shinnar S. Long-term cognitive outcomes of a cohort of children with cryptogenic infantile spasms treated with high-dose adrenocorticotropic hormone. *Epilepsia* 2004; 45: 255-62.

Klein R, Livingston S. The effect of adrenocorticotropic hormone in epilepsy. *J Pediatr* 1950; 37: 733-42.

Kondo Y, Okumura A, Watanabe K, *et al.* Comparison of two low dose ACTH therapies for West syndrome: their efficacy and side effect. *Brain Dev* 2005; 27: 326-30.

Kossoff EH, Pyzik PL, McGrogan JR, Vining EP, Freeman JM. Efficacy of the ketogenic diet for infantile spasms. *Pediatrics* 2002; 109: 780-3.

Kusse MC, van Nieuwenhuizen O, van Huffelen AC, van der Mey W, Thijssen JH, van Ree JM. The effect of non-depot ACTH(1-24) on infantile spasms. *Dev Med Child Neurol* 1993; 35: 1067-73.

Lagae L, Buyse G, Deconinck A, Ceulemans B. Effect of levetiracetam in refractory childhood epilepsy syndromes. *Eur J Paediatr Neurol* 2003; 7: 123-8.

Lawlor KM, Devlin AM. Levetiracetam in the treatment of infantile spasms. *Eur J Paediatr Neurol* 2005; 9: 19-22.

Lee WS, Limmroth V, Ayata C *et al.*. Peripheral GABAA receptor-mediated effects of sodium valproate on dural plasma protein extravasation to substance P and trigeminal stimulation. *Br J Pharmacol* 1995; 116: 1661-7.

Lerman P, Kivity S. The efficacy of corticotropin in primary infantile spasms. *J Pediatr* 1982; 101: 294-6.

Lombroso CT. A prospective study of infantile spasms: clinical and therapeutic correlations. *Epilepsia*. 1983; 24: 135-58.

Lotze TE, Wilfong AA. Zonisamide treatment for symptomatic infantile spasms. *Neurology* 2004; 62: 296-8.

Lux AL, Edwards SW, Hancock E *et al.* The United Kingdom Infantile Spasms Study comparing vigabatrin with prednisolone or tetracosactide at 14 days: a multicentre, randomised controlled trial. *Lancet* 2004; 364: 1773-8.

Lux AL, Edwards SW, Hancock E et al. The United Kingdom Infantile Spasms Study (UKISS) comparing hormone treatment with vigabatrin on developmental and epilepsy outcomes to age 14 months: a multicentre randomised trial. *Lancet Neurol* 2005; 4: 712-7.

Mackay MT, Weiss SK, Adams-Webber T et al. Practice parameter: medical treatment of infantile spasms: report of the American Academy of Neurology and the Child Neurology Society. *Neurology* 2004; 62: 1668-81.

Matsuishi T, Yano E, Inanaga K, et al. A pilot study on the anticonvulsive effects of a thyrotropin-releasing hormone analog in intractable epilepsy. *Brain Dev* 1983; 5: 421-8.

Matsumoto A, Kumagai T, Takeuchi T et al. Clinical effects of thyrotropin-releasing hormone for severe epilepsy in childhood: a comparative study with ACTH therapy. *Epilepsia* 1987; 28: 49-55.

Matsumoto A, Kumagai T, Takeuchi T et al. Factors influencing effectiveness of thyrotropin-releasing hormone therapy for severe epilepsy in childhood: significance of serum prolactin levels. *Epilepsia*. 1989; 30: 45-9.

Matsumoto A, Watanabe K, Negoro T, et al. Long-term prognosis after infantile spasms: a statistical study of prognostic factors in 200 cases. *Dev Med Child Neurol* 1981; 23: 51-65.

Mikaeloff Y, de Saint-Martin A, Mancini J et al. Topiramate: efficacy and tolerability in children according to epilepsy syndromes. *Epilepsy Res* 2003; 53: 225-32.

Mikati MA, Fayad M, Koleilat M et al. Efficacy, tolerability, and kinetics of lamotrigine in infants. *J Pediatr* 2002; 141: 31-5.

Montelli TC, Mota NG, Peracoli MT, Torres EA, Rezkallah-Iwasso MT. Immunological disturbance in West and Lennox-Gastaut syndromes. *Arq Neuropsiquiatr* 1984; 42: 132-9.

Mota NG, Rezkallah-Iwasso MT, Peracoli MT, Montelli TC. Demonstration of antibody and cellular immune response to brain extract in West and Lennox-Gastaut syndromes. *Arq Neuropsiquiatr* 1984; 42: 126-31.

Nordli DR J, rKuroda MM, Carroll J, et al. Experience with the ketogenic diet in infants. *Pediatrics*. 2001; 108 (1): 129-33.

Oguni H, Funatsuka M, Sasaki K et al. Effect of ACTH therapy for epileptic spasms without hypsarrhythmia. *Epilepsia*. 2005; 46: 709-15.

Oguni H, Yanagaki S, Hayashi K et al. Extremely low-dose ACTH step-up protocol for West syndrome: maximum therapeutic effect with minimal side effects. *Brain Dev* 2006; 28: 8-13.

Ohtsuka Y, Matsuda M, Ogino T et al. Treatment of the West syndrome with high-dose pyridoxal phosphate. *Brain Dev* 1987; 9: 418-21.

Perucca E, Dulac O, Shorvon S, Tomson T. Harnessing the clinical potential of antiepileptic drug therapy: dosage optimisation. *CNS Drugs* 2001; 15: 609-21.

Pietz J, Benninger C, Schafer H, Sontheimer D, Mittermaier G, Rating D. Treatment of infantile spasms with high-dosage vitamin B6. *Epilepsia* 1993; 34: 757-63.

Riikonen R. A long-term follow-up study of 214 children with the syndrome of infantile spasms. *Neuropediatrics* 1982; 13: 14-23.

Riikonen R. Infantile spasms: modern practical aspects. *Acta Paediatr Scand* 1984; 73: ???.

Rubenstein JE, Kossoff EH, Pyzik PL, Vining EP, McGrogan JR, Freeman JM. Experience in the use of the ketogenic diet as early therapy. *J Child Neurol* 2005; 20: 31-4.

Shields D. Medical *versus* surgical treatment: which treatment when. In *"Epilepsy, Infantile Spasms and Developmental Encephalopathy."* Ed. By P. Schwrtzkhroin and J.Rho. Academic Press, 2002: 253-65.

Siemes H, Brandl U, Spohr HL, Volger S, Weschke B. Long-term follow-up study of vigabatrin in pretreated children with West syndrome. *Seizure* 1998; 7: 293-7.

Siemes H, Siegert M, Aksu F, Emrich R, Hanefeld F, Scheffner D. CSF protein profile in infantile spasms. Influence of etiology and ACTH or dexamethasone treatment. *Epilepsia* 1984; 25: 368-76.

Snead OC 3rd, Benton JW Jr, Hosey LC et al. Treatment of infantile spasms with high-dose ACTH: efficacy and plasma levels of ACTH and cortisol. *Neurology* 1989; 39: 1027-31.

Snead OC 3rd, Benton JW, Myers GJ. ACTH and prednisone in childhood seizure disorders. *Neurology* 1983; 33: 966-70.

Sorel L,Dusaucy-Bauloye A. Findings in 21 cases of Gibbs' hypsarrhythmia; spectacular effectiveness of ACTH.] *Acta Neurol Psychiatr Belg.* 1958; 58: 130-41.

Suzuki Y, Nagai T, Ono J et al. Zonisamide monotherapy in newly diagnosed infantile spasms. *Epilepsia* 1997; 38: 1035-8.

Takeuchi Y, Takano T, Abe J et al. Thyrotropin-releasing hormone: role in the treatment of West syndrome and related epileptic encephalopathies. *Brain Dev* 2001; 23: 662-7.

Takeuchi Y, Tominaga M, Mitsufuji N, et al. Thyrotropin-releasing hormone in treatment of intractable epilepsy: neurochemical analysis of CSF monoamine metabolites *Pediatr Neurol* 1995; 12: 139-45.

Takuma Y. ACTH therapy for infantile spasms: a combination therapy with high-dose pyridoxal phosphate and low-dose ACTH. *Epilepsia* 1998; 39 (suppl 5): 42-5.

Thijs J, Verhelst H, Van Coster R. Retrospective study of topiramate in a paediatric population with intractable epilepsy showing promising effects in the West syndrome patients. *Acta Neurol Belg* 2001; 101: 171-6.

van Engelen BG, Renier WO, Weemaes CM, Strengers PF, Bernsen PJ, Notermans SL. High-dose intravenous immunoglobulin treatment in cryptogenic West and Lennox-Gastaut syndrome; an add-on study. *Eur J Pediatr.* 1994; 153: 762-9.

Vassella F, Pavlincova E, Schneider HJ, Rudin HJ, Karbowski K. Treatment of infantile spasms and Lennox-Gastaut syndrome with clonazepam (Rivotril). *Epilepsia.* 1973; 14: 165-75.

Veggiotti P, Cieuta C, Rex E, Dulac O. Lamotrigine in infantile spasms. *Lancet.* 1994; 344: 1375-6.

Vigevano F, Cilio MR. Vigabatrin *versus* ACTH as first-line treatment for infantile spasms: a randomized, prospective study. *Epilepsia.* 1997; 38: 1270-4.

Vles JS, van der Heyden AM, Ghijs A, Troost J. Vigabatrin in the treatment of infantile spasms. *Neuropediatrics.* 1993; 24: 230-1.

Yanagaki S, Oguni H, Hayashi K et al. A comparative study of high-dose and low-dose ACTH therapy for West syndrome. *Brain Dev* 1999; 2: 461-7.

Yanai S, Hanai T, Narazaki O. Treatment of infantile spasms with zonisamide. *Brain Dev* 1999; 21: 157-61.

Achevé d'imprimer par Corlet, Imprimeur, S.A.
14110 Condé-sur-Noireau
N° d'Imprimeur : 99666 - Dépôt légal : juin 2007
Imprimé en France